Quantitative Methods in Social Work: State of the Art

Quantitative Methods in Social Work: State of the Art

David F. Gillespie
Charles Glisson
Editors

The Haworth Press, Inc.
New York • London • Norwood (Australia)

Quantitative Methods in Social Work: State of the Art has also been published as the *Journal of Social Service Research*, Volume 16, Numbers 1/2 1992.

© 1992 by The Haworth Press, Inc. All rights reserved. No part of this work may be reproduced or utilized in any form or by any means, electronic or mechanical, including photocopying, microfilm and recording, or by any information storage and retrieval system, without permission in writing from the publisher. Printed in the United States of America.

The Haworth Press, Inc., 10 Alice Street, Binghamton, NY 13904-1580 USA

Library of Congress Cataloging-in-Publication Data

Quantitative methods in social work : state of the art / David F. Gillespie, Charles Glisson, editors.
      p. cm.
  Includes bibliographical references and index.
  ISBN 1-56024-274-4.–ISBN 1-56024-275-2 (pbk.)
   1. Social service–Statistical methods. I. Gillespie, David F. II. Glisson, Charles.
HV29.Q36 1992
001.4'22'024362–dc20   92-29647
                                                                                          CIP

Quantitative Methods in Social Work: State of the Art

CONTENTS

Toward the Development of Quantitative Methods
   in Social Work Research   1
      Charles Glisson
      David F. Gillespie

A Comparison of Classical, Item Response,
   and Generalizability Theories of Measurement   11
      William R. Nugent
      Janette A. Hankins

Using the Computer for Content Analysis   41
      Jane C. Kronick
      Susan Silver

A Preliminary Examination of the Knowledge
   of Normative Infant Development (KNID) Inventory
   Using Structural Equation Modeling   59
      John G. Orme
      Judith Ann Fickling

The Use of Logistic Regression in Social Work Research   87
      Nancy Morrow-Howell
      Enola K. Proctor

Loglinear Analysis in Social Work Research   105
      Terri Combs-Orme

Event History Analysis: A Proportional Hazards Perspective on Modeling Outcomes in Intensive Family Preservation Services 123
    Mark W. Fraser
    Peter J. Pecora
    Chirapat Popuang
    David A. Haapala

Moderator Variables in Social Work Research 159
    Gary F. Koeske

Interaction Effects in Multiple Regression 179
    Claudia Coulton
    Julian Chow

Social Network Analysis 201
    Calvin L. Streeter
    David F. Gillespie

Index 223

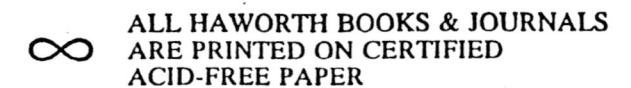

∞ ALL HAWORTH BOOKS & JOURNALS ARE PRINTED ON CERTIFIED ACID-FREE PAPER

ABOUT THE EDITORS

David F. Gillespie earned his PhD in Sociology from the University of Washington in Seattle. He is currently Professor of Social Work at the George Warren Brown School of Social Work, Washington University in St. Louis. He has undertaken studies for a number of non-profit and private organizations, including the National Science Foundation, the Health, Education and Welfare Department, the American Red Cross, and Union Electric Company. His current research is funded by the National Science Foundation and concentrates on the American Red Cross and its network of interorganizational relations for disaster preparedness. He has published several books and numerous papers on organizations and research methodology.

Charles Glisson earned his PhD in Social Work from Washington University in St. Louis. He is currently Professor and Chair, PhD Program in Social Work, College of Social Work, University of Tennessee-Knoxville. His current research is a three year NIMH R01 Research Grant studying the interorganizational coordination of services to children in state custody. He has published numerous chapters and articles on social work research methodology, services research, and human service organizations.

Quantitative Methods in Social Work: State of the Art

Toward the Development of Quantitative Methods in Social Work Research

Charles Glisson
David F. Gillespie

The following paragraph describes the medical care received by Charles II of England in 1685.

A pint of blood was extracted from his right arm; then eight ounces from the left shoulder; next an emetic, two physics, and an enema consisting of 15 substances. Then his head was shaved and a blister raised on the scalp. To purge the brain a sneezing powder was given, then cowslip powder to strengthen it. Meanwhile more emetics, soothing drinks and more bleeding; also a plaster of pitch and pigeon dung applied to the royal feet. Not to leave anything undone, the following substances were taken internally: melon seeds, manna, slippery elm, black cherry water, extract of lily of the valley, peony, lavender, pearls dissolved in vinegar, gentian root, nutmeg, and finally 40 drops of extract of human skull. As a last resort, bezoar stone was employed. But the royal patient died. (MacKinney, 1937:33)

Because he was a member of the royal family, Charles II received what was thought to be the best medical treatment available. Certainly, commoners could not have hoped for such intensive medical attention. Of course they were undoubtedly better off for it since many deaths can now be traced directly to the treatments. In fact, until about 1900, calling in a physician to attend the sick appears to have decreased the patient's chances for survival (Hardin, 1972: 57-58). It wasn't until medical research demonstrated the effectiveness of sulfa drugs in the 1930's and antibiotics in the 1940's that medical treatment began to

---

Charles Glisson is Professor and Chair, PhD Program, College of Social Work, University of Tennessee, Knoxville, TN 37996. David F. Gillespie is Professor, George Warren Brown School of Social Work, Washington University, St. Louis, MO 63130.

The authors appreciate the comments and suggestions made by Susan A. Murty on an earlier version of this paper.

Requests for reprints should be sent to Charles Glisson, College of Social Work, University of Tennessee, Knoxville, TN 37996.

© 1992 by The Haworth Press, Inc. All rights reserved.

increase significantly a patient's chances of survival. Today, morbidity and mortality rates are generally reduced with appropriate and timely medical care.

Contemporary social work practice may not resemble the antiquated medical care of the 1600's. Yet much of what social workers do must be accepted on the type of faith that guided the treatment of Charles II. Critics accuse social work practitioners of relying on interventions which are ineffective and in some cases harmful. Moreover, social work research efforts have failed to quell doubts concerning social work interventions. Even the staunchest defenders of social work research would not claim that it has contributed significantly to or documented convincingly the effectiveness of practice. There are multiple reasons for this, some related to the nature of the problems addressed by social workers, some related to the training received by social workers, and some related to the deficits in the research conducted by social workers.

The deficits in social work research efforts to establish practice efficacy are addressed here. The deficits are both theoretical and methodological in origin. Social science research and more recently social work research have become increasingly empirically grounded. Unfortunately, it is for this reason that data collection and data analysis have become all too often the central activities of social science research. Because of this, critics have chided social work researchers for their failure to conduct research which is oriented to practice issues and of addressing technical or scientific concerns which have little direct relevance to practice. Social work researchers have also been taken to task by their colleagues for neglecting to link their research findings with substantive theories, and for collecting data and running analyses without any firm research purpose in mind. These criticisms call for a careful critique of the state of the art of social work research, and in particular an examination of the contributions of theory and method to the practice relevance of research outcomes.

Most scientific research rests on the relationship between substantive theory and methods of inquiry. Unfortunately, the separation of substance and method is more characteristic of the social sciences than of the physical sciences. For example, it is common for research methods to be discussed as an integral part of the substantive content of textbooks in biology and physics. This blending of method and substance occurs, in part, because research and theory development in these sciences are approached as puzzle-solving (Kuhn, 1962; Laudan, 1977). In other words, these sciences view theory as derived from solving puzzles (i.e., problems) and view research methods as essential to solving the puzzles. As a result, substantive areas are not addressed analytically apart from the methods used to solve the relevant puzzles.

Social work texts are devoted more often than not to either substantive theory or to research methodology that is devoid of substantive applications. This separation of substantive theory and research methodology has contributed to a breach between what should be inseparable parts of the research process. More emphasis on puzzle or problem-solving in social work research could help bridge the gap between substance and method and also help deal with some of the issues dividing researchers and practitioners. However, this problem-solving approach requires a greater appreciation and understanding of research methods by social work practitioners. Likewise, this approach also requires a greater appreciation and understanding of substantive practice areas by social work researchers.

The suggestion that social work researchers become more involved in practice while practitioners become more knowledgeable of research methods has become a common platitude and may be viewed as desirable but unrealistic given the intense and continuous demands on each of these roles (Austin, 1991). On the other hand, recent trends indicate the possibility of a convergence. First, the rapidly spreading use of micro computers in both practice and social work research provide a common link in the way information is processed. Second, the emphasis on accountability and evaluation is creating the need in the practice community for information which can be used to solve problems. Third, menu driven software is rendering sophisticated methodological techniques accessible to the beginning problem or puzzle-solver. Still, it is clear that social work research is in a neophyte stage and that considerable work is needed before social workers will be able to produce a substantial body of relevant, high-quality research that contributes directly to the solution of the most critical puzzles and problems which social workers face in their practice.

NIMH TASK FORCE ON SOCIAL WORK RESEARCH

By forming the NIMH Task Force on Social Work Research, the National Institute of Mental Health can be credited with beginning one of the first nationally organized efforts to improve social work research. The Task Force recently completed a three-year effort to understand why so few social work researchers are among the social, behavioral and biological scientists who are supported by NIMH to conduct mental health-related research. The Task Force found evidence that social work researchers do not have the research skills to compete successfully for research funding. Reports commissioned by the Task Force document deficiencies in both the quality of social work research training and the quality of published social work research.

In one report commissioned by the Task Force, Glisson (1990) summarizes the social work research published over a twelve-year period. The report is based on an analysis of all of the research articles published from 1977 through 1988 in five major social work journals: *Journal of Social Service Research, Journal of Social Work Education, Social Service Review, Social Work,* and *Social Work Research and Abstracts.* The findings provide a description of the underdeveloped state of social work research and point to several problems confronting efforts to develop research-based knowledge for social work. A parallel study commissioned by the Task Force to examine additional journals reports similar findings (Fraser and Taylor, 1990).

A summary of some of the findings of the Glisson (1990) report are provided below as an introduction to a discussion of the development of quantitative methods in social work research. The report defines research broadly. An article is considered research-based if the author bases conclusions on any type of systematic observations. This includes case studies, field studies, historical research, and single subject research, as well as survey, experimental and quasi-experimental research. Of the almost two thousand articles published in the five journals from 1977 through 1988, only a little more than half (1,053) can be labeled research-based using this broad definition. Both the numbers and the proportions of research articles published in these journals annually have remained stubbornly consistent, averaging 90 (53%) per year in the first six-year period and 85 (56%) per year in the second six-year period. In contrast, there is considerable variation between the individual journals in the proportions of published articles that are research-based. The proportions range from a high of 83% in the *Journal of Social Service Research* to a low of 39% in *Social Work*.

While the overall numbers and proportions of research articles published in the five journals have remained consistent over the twelve-year period, there are several trends evident in the research articles themselves. The more positive trends include an increased emphasis in the articles on effectiveness and outcome variables. Such research almost doubled from 27% of the research articles published in the first six years (1977-1982) to 52% of the research articles published in the second six years (1983-1988). This increase suggests the development of a greater practice orientation in research as social work scholars have become increasingly concerned with documenting effectiveness and outcomes (Austin, 1991).

A parallel trend has been the increase in the number of research articles that are concerned specifically with direct practice, particularly with individuals. In the last six years, half of the research articles concerned direct practice and 40% concerned direct practice with individuals. The heightened focus on direct practice with individuals stems partly from professional ideology and partly from the current disproportionate influence of psychology on social work practice and research. Although historically social work has drawn upon sociology, economics, political science, and other more macro-oriented social science disciplines, social work and psychology appear to be increasingly competing in the same practice arena for the same clients and in the same research arena for the same research funding, as found in the funding provided by NIMH.

Among the more negative findings concerning social work research is the steady dominance throughout the twelve-year period of quick, inexpensive and relatively simple research methods. Cross-sectional survey designs are reported in the majority of the research articles (63%). The design which is reported next most often is the case study (13%), followed by the quasi-experimental design (9%). In addition, 74% of the articles report research that relies on nonrepresentative samples of convenience. Moreover, while 85% of the articles rely on some type of quantitative analysis, half of these articles report only descriptive statistics such as percentages and means, or univariate statistics that incorporate only one independent and one dependent variable at a time. The risk of inferential error is high when these simplistic statistical techniques are coupled with the low internal validity and low external validity of the research strategies reported in these articles. This risk is particularly serious when inferences are being drawn about practice effectiveness and outcomes as is the case in half of the research articles published in the last six-year period.

Despite some of these negative findings, there is also evident a small but increasing concern in this literature with the further development of social work research methods. In 8% of the articles published in the last six-year period, attention is given specifically to the development of social work research methods. Moreover, the proportion of research articles incorporating more sophisticated multivariate data analytic techniques almost doubled from the first six years (8.7%) to the second six years (16.2%). There is, therefore, evidence that social work researchers are beginning to be interested in developing more sophisticated research methods and to incorporate more powerful analytic techniques in their research. The attraction of these more advanced methods and techniques is that they improve the researcher's ability to study complex social problems and interventions while reducing the risk of oversimplification and inferential error.

IMPLICATIONS OF THE NIMH REPORT FINDINGS

There are symbiotic relationships among three key aspects of the social work research effort. These are the social work researchers themselves, the social work doctoral programs which train them, and the social work research literature in which their work is published. The characteristics of each of these aspects informs and affects the other two. Glisson's (1990) report documents that the vast majority of the social work research literature is produced by those who have social work doctorates or are members of social work program faculties. Therefore, inadequacies identified in existing social work research are to some extent maintained in a "cycle of poverty" of knowledge: poorly trained researchers produce poor research and poorly trained researchers who, in turn, produce more poor research and more poorly trained researchers.

The evidence provided in the report confirms Glisson's previous findings concerning poor statistical training received by social workers (Glisson and Fischer, 1987) and the inadequate application of statistical analyses in published social work research (Glisson, 1985). Because the more sophisticated analytic techniques are currently found in only about 16% of the research articles and because the research articles represent only about half of the articles published in the major social work journals, it can be assumed that knowledge of sophisticated methods among social work researchers remains limited.

These conclusions suggest the need for more information concerning the levels of expertise among those who are developing and using social work research knowledge. This also suggests the need for more widespread dissemination of existing research-based knowledge to social work researchers. Until there is a broader understanding and application of more sophisticated methods throughout the social work literature, we are unlikely to achieve research which will be useful in solving the most complex and critical problems facing social work practice.

A RESPONSE TO THE NEED

A group of social work researchers has recognized the need for a broader understanding and application of advanced research methods among social work researchers generally. Some three years ago, this group emerged to form the Quantitative Methods Interest Group (QMIG) for the purpose of developing and disseminating knowledge about the application of quantitative analytic techniques in social work research. Each year since its founding, the QMIG has sponsored a Quantitative Methods Symposium at the Council on Social Work Education Annual Program Meeting. In addition, the QMIG has compiled the papers in this collection, most of which were written by members of the interest group. The papers are intended to give examples of the most advanced research now being carried out in the profession in various areas of knowledge relevant to the field of social work. It is also intended that they will stimulate the further development of quantitative methodology among social work researchers.

The authors of the papers presented here assume that the reader is familiar with basic research methodology, including descriptive statistics and the elementary inferential statistics used most often in published social work research: t-tests, analysis of variance, and correlation/regression techniques. The papers address several significant methodological issues involved in using quantitative analytic techniques that are state-of-the-art for social work research. In most cases, the techniques are state-of-the-art in other disciplines as well, although in some papers the techniques are presented in their basic forms. This is consistent with the goal of stimulating the development of more advanced quantitative methods in social work research.

Three types of methodological issues are addressed in the papers: (1) measurement issues; (2) issues related to incorporating non-quantitative variables in quantitative data analyses; and (3) issues surrounding the use of quantitative analytic techniques to model and assess complex social phenomena. An elaboration of each of these three issues is presented below. Although the content of some of the papers overlaps more than one of these issues, they are grouped by the primary issue that is addressed.

Measurement

As in the social sciences generally, measurement issues in social work research are particularly problematic. Many of the variables that are of concern to social worker researchers are abstract constructs that are not easy to observe directly. Examples are self-esteem, depression and marital satisfaction measured at the individual level; cohesion, cooperation and participation at the group level; complexity, centralization and formalization at the organizational level; and stratification, power and oppression at the societal level. Attempts to assess such variables and estimate their accuracy are plagued with difficulties, yet very little work has been completed to date among social work researchers concerning measurement (see Hudson, 1982, for an exception).

The paper by Nugent and Hankins compares the application of the three major theories of measurement–classical, generalizability, and item response theories– to the evaluation of Hudson's (1982) Generalized Contentment Scale (GCS), an instrument that is used by both social work researchers and practitioners to measure depression. The paper compares the different types of measurement information provided by the three approaches and describes the strengths and weaknesses of each. In contrast, the paper by Kronick and Silver describes content analysis, a technique that is usually not considered a measurement technique, and applies it to the study of health policy using the Canada Health Act as an example. Content analysis is a method for identifying and measuring the occurrence of concepts, phrases, and other variables within the content of documents, transcripts, interviews and group interactions. The paper compares the utility of several software packages that can be used in content analyses and provides practical suggestions for improving their applications. The third measurement paper, by Orme and Fickling, illustrates the use of latent variable structural equation modeling (LISREL) in assessing the validity of a scale that is designed to measure a parent's knowledge of infant development. LISREL has continued to become more and more popular among social science researchers for confirming measurement models as well as for analyzing the structure of complex relationships among multiple exogenous and endogenous variables. Since applications of LISREL in social work research are rare, this paper makes an important contribution to this volume.

Incorporating Qualitative Variables into Quantitative Analyses

There are many methods for incorporating into quantitative analytic techniques variables which are commonly labeled nominal, categorical or qualitative. Analysis of variance is designed specifically for these types of independent variables. Qualitative variables also can be easily included in correlation/ regression analyses with the aid of special coding. In addition to these relatively common methods, there are other powerful analytic techniques designed specifically for qualitative variables; unfortunately these are used much less frequently by social work researchers. For example, logistic regression is designed for the analysis of qualitative dependent variables, loglinear analysis is designed for both qualitative independent and qualitative dependent variables, and event history analysis provides for the longitudinal analysis of a specific type of qualitative dependent variable, the occurrence of an event.

These three techniques, logistic regression, loglinear analysis and event history analysis, are described and applied in separate papers in this collection. Morrow-Howell and Proctor demonstrate the use of logistic regression in their research on the factors contributing to hospital readmissions among Medicare patients. Combs-Orme explains the application of log-linear analysis using examples from published social work studies of alcoholism and minority adolescent parents. Fraser, Pecora, Popuang and Haapala demonstrate the use of event history analysis in identifying the factors that contribute to the success or failure of family preservation services. These techniques have special significance to social work researchers because so many substantive and practice-related variables are qualitative in nature.

Modeling Complex Social Phenomena

Social work research is frequently concerned with complex social phenomena which cannot be accurately represented by simple bivariate relationships or by a collection of main effects. For example, moderator effects occur when the effect of one variable on another is contingent upon the values of a third variable. Koeske uses studies of worker burnout and income bias to describe a variety of moderation effects which, if ignored or unanalyzed, can pose threats to the validity of findings. In a related paper, Coulton and Chow use studies of depression and locus of control to describe the analysis of interactions using regression techniques that include continuous moderator variables rather than the more traditional categorical moderator variables.

Another example of complex social phenomena of interest to social work researchers is the nature of networks or relations among multiple social units. Whether the relationships describe networks of individuals, as in a family, or networks of organizations or other larger social units, depicting and analyzing the structure of relationships and their consequences can be frustrating if not impossible with the usual analytic approaches. Network analysis has been used with increasing frequency in anthropology and sociology to describe and understand complex networks, but is used infrequently in social work. Streeter and Gillespie present a basic explanation of network analysis and apply it to social service organizational networks that respond to natural disasters.

Many complex phenomena of interest to social work researchers are events that occur at different times for different members of a population of interest. These include events such as marriages, divorces, residential placements, spouse abuse, adoptions, recidivism, and so forth. Although used more often by biostatisticians, sociologists, and economists than by social work researchers, event history analysis has been developed specifically for analyzing these types of phenomena with longitudinal data. As mentioned above, the paper by Fraser et al., describes the theoretical foundations of the method and provides an example by using event history analysis to identify factors that prevent or contribute to the out-of-home placement of children who participate in family preservation programs.

RELATED ISSUES

There are numerous issues related to quantitative methods in social work research that have not been addressed by the papers in this collection. These include issues of sampling and design, as well as additional issues surrounding measurement and data analysis. Several related multivariate analytic techniques that provide for the simultaneous analysis of multiple independent and multiple dependent variables are not considered here. These multivariate techniques include canonical analysis, multivariate analysis of variance, and multivariate multiple regression. Although the use of LISREL is described in the context of assessing a measurement model, its use in analyzing more complex structural equation models is not described. Finally, still other quantitative methods that are applied with increasing frequency in social work research are missing from this collection, including time-series analysis and meta-analysis.

The omission of papers that address these additional issues and methods is not intentional and is not intended to suggest that they are less important than those which have been included. Rather, it suggests that the major objectives of the present collection cannot be fully met with one volume. There is a need for subsequent similar collections.

At the same time, the articles that follow are successful in describing several distinct and effective strategies used by social work researchers in addressing three critical methodological issues within specific substantive contexts. These articles collectively represent some of the best research efforts currently found among social workers and provide both a guide and a challenge to social work researchers interested in the application of quantitative methods to social work problem-solving.

REFERENCES

Austin, David. 1991. "Comments on Research Development in Social Work." *Social Work Research & Abstracts* 27(1):38-41.

Fraser, Mark, and Mary Jane Taylor. 1990. "An Assessment of the Literature in Social Work." Commissioned by the National Institute of Mental Health Task Force on Social Work Research.

Glisson, Charles. 1985. "In Defense of Statistical Tests of Significance." *Social Service Review* 59(3):377-386.

Glisson, Charles. 1990. "A Systematic Assessment of the Social Work Literature: Trends in Social Work Research." Commissioned by the National Institute of Mental Health Task Force on Social Work Research.

Glisson, Charles, and Joel Fischer. 1987. "Statistical Training for Social Workers." *Journal of Social Work Education* 23(3):50-58.

Hardin, Garrett James. 1973. *Stalking the Wild Taboo*. Los Altos, California: William Kaufmann, Inc.

Kuhn, Thomas S. 1962. *The Structure of Scientific Revolutions*. Chicago: The University of Chicago Press.

Laudan, Larry. 1977. *Progress and its Problems*. Berkeley: University of California Press.

MacKinney, Loren C. 1937. *Early Medieval Medicine with Special Reference to France and Chartres*. Baltimore: The Johns Hopkins Press.

A Comparison of Classical, Item Response, and Generalizability Theories of Measurement

William R. Nugent
Janette A. Hankins

SUMMARY. This article compares important concepts from Classical Measurement Theory, Item Response Theory, and Generalizability Theory. A brief, somewhat technical overview of each of these measurement theories is given. Important conceptual and technical similarities and differences between each of these theories are then noted. Several hundred responses on Hudson's Generalized Contentment Scale are analyzed using each of these measurement theories and the results used to illustrate

---

William R. Nugent received his PhD in Social Work from Florida State University. He is currently with the College of Social Work, University of Tennessee. He is involved in research on applied measurement in assessment; on the effects of different verbal interventions on clients during social work interviews; and on methods for integrating single case design and group comparison methodologies for practice evaluation. He has recently published an article on the psychometric characteristics of self-anchored scales: Nugent, W.R., Hankins, J.A. (1989). The use of item response theory in social work measurement and research. *Social Service Review, 63*, 447-473.

Janette A. Hankins received her PhD in Educational Measurement and Testing from Florida State University in 1986. She is currently with the Office of Public Service, University of Tennessee. She is doing research on adaptive testing and on procedures for setting cut scores on criterion referenced tests. She has recently published an article on adaptive testing: Hankins, J.A. (1990). The effects of variable entry for a bayesian adaptive test. *Educational and Psychological Measurement, 50*, 785-802; and co-authored an article with Bill Nugent: Nugent, W.R., Hankins, J.A. (1989). The use of item response theory in social work measurement and research. *Social Service Review, 63*, 447-473.

Requests for reprints should be sent to William R. Nugent, College of Social Work, University of Tennessee, Knoxville, TN 37996.

© 1992 by The Haworth Press, Inc. All rights reserved.

concepts from, and similarities and differences between, each of these theories.

Measurement is a fundamental and critical aspect of social research. Poor measurement can render useless otherwise well conceived and executed research. Further, as expressed by Nunnally (1978, p. 6), ". . . major advances in psychology, and probably in all sciences, are preceded by breakthroughs in measurement methods."

Numerous evaluation and research texts contain elementary chapters on measurement (e.g., Kerlinger, 1973) as do some practice oriented works (e.g., Hudson, 1982). These works describe various aspects of Classical Measurement Theory, perhaps the most commonly used measurement theory in the social sciences. Social work researchers also rely on Classical Measurement Theory. For example, the scales contained in Hudson's (1982) and Corcoran and Fischer's (1987) works are based on principles of Classical Theory. However, there are two alternate theories which have received increasing attention in other disciplines, but have been essentially ignored in social work research: Item Response Theory (IRT) and Generalizability Theory. In many ways these theories are more powerful and have broader application than Classical theory, allowing the researcher to do things that would otherwise not be possible, such as adaptive testing and the multifacet analysis of measurement error.

This article compares and contrasts aspects of Classical, Item Response, and Generalizability theories. First, the breakdown of scores in each of these theories is discussed. Next, the concept of reliability in each theory is elaborated and important similarities and differences in these theories are described. Analyses of responses on Hudson's Generalized Contentment Scale (GCS), a 25-item Likert Type scale that is used by many social work practitioners and researchers to measure non-psychotic depression (Hudson, 1982), are used to illustrate applications of each of the measurement theories described.[1] For the reader unfamiliar with these theories, the following provide excellent coverage and introductions: Classical theory (Nunnally, 1978; Ghiselli, Campbell, & Zedeck, 1981; Allen & Yen, 1979); Item Response Theory (Warm, 1978; Lord, 1980; Hambleton & Swamanathan, 1985); Generalizability Theory (Cronbach, Gleser, Nanda, & Rajaratnam, 1972; Brennan, 1983; Shavelson, Webb, & Rowley, 1989). Crocker and Algina (1986) give an excellent introduction to each theory.

SCORE BREAKDOWN

Classical Theory

In Classical theory an observed score, X, is broken down into two components: a true score, T, and an error score, E:

$$X = T + E. \tag{1}$$

The true score, a fundamental concept in Classical theory, is defined as:

$$\varepsilon(X) = T, \tag{2}$$

where ε = the "expectation" operator.

That is, the true score on a given measurement is the expected value (mean) of the observed score X over a very large number of parallel measurements. The error score E lumps the effects of all sources of error into a single undifferentiated term (Lord & Novick, 1968; Crocker & Algina, 1986). Equation (1) leads to the Classical variance breakdown,

$$\sigma^2(X) = \sigma^2(T) + \sigma^2(E). \tag{3}$$

Item Response Theory

In Item Response Theory (IRT), an important assumption states that the probability of an individual responding to a given item in a given manner, $p(\theta)$, is a monotonic increasing function *only* of the individual's level of the trait measured by the item.[2] The trait that underlies the individual's response is scaled on a continuous metric called the theta (θ) metric, with values of θ ranging from $+\infty$ to $-\infty$. The nonlinear relationship between the response and the metric θ is called an *item response function* (IRF) or *item characteristic curve* (ICC) (Hambleton & Swamanathan, 1985). The mathematical form of the two parameter logistic (2PL) IRF is:

$$p_g(\theta) = \frac{1}{1 + e^{-1.7\, a_g(\theta - b_g)}}, \tag{4}$$

where $p_g(\theta)$ = the probability that item g is scored with a 1,
e = the base of the natural logarithms,
a_g = the *a* value for item g,
and b_g = the *b* value for item g.

The *a* value is the "item discrimination" index and is related to the maximum slope of the IRF (Lord, 1980). The *a* value is a measure of the degree to which item response varies with trait level and is an indicator of the maximum discrimination between different θ levels given by the item. The *b* value is the "item difficulty" index. It gives the θ value at which the probability that an item is positively endorsed is 0.5, and it gives the location on the θ scale at which the slope of the IRF is maximum and thus discriminates maximally between different θ levels (Lord, 1980).

If the response to item g is u_g, then, since the IRF is the regression of item response on θ, $\varepsilon(u_g \mid \theta) = p_g(\theta)$ (Hambleton & Swamanathan, 1985). In Classical theory, $\varepsilon(u_g \mid \theta) = T$, where T is the true score. Thus, $p_g(\theta) = T$ and so θ is the same thing as item true score except for the scale on which they are measured (Lord, 1980; Hambleton & Swamanathan, 1985). A critical difference between the true score metric and the θ metric, however, is that the true score is item dependent, where the θ metric is not (Lord, 1980).

The *test characteristic function*, $T(\theta)$, is the regression of X on θ and relates true score over a set of n items to the θ metric (Warm, 1978; Lord, 1980):

$$T(\theta) = \sum_{g=1}^{n} p_g(\theta) = \varepsilon(X \mid \theta) \tag{5}$$

Thus, the breakdown of an observed score X in IRT is given by,

$$X = \sum_{g=1}^{n} p_g(\theta) + E = T + E, \tag{6}$$

where E is the error term (Crocker & Algina, 1986). As in Classical theory, the error component lumps all sources of error into a single undifferentiated term.

Generalizability Theory

In Generalizability, or G-theory the researcher is concerned with inferring the characteristics of a much larger set of measurements from measurements taken under certain specific conditions. Consider the person-by-item matrix in Figure 1 in which there is an infinite number of persons from a population, P, who have responded to each of an infinite number of items. Each cell in the matrix contains a response by a person to an item. The infinite set of items comprises a universe of items that is called a *facet* of measurement. A facet is any condition of a measurement procedure. The set of all possible admissible conditions of measurement is called the *universe of admissible observations*. The infinite set of responses in the matrix in Figure 1 represents the responses of all persons in P to all conditions (i.e., items) in the universe of admissible observations for this single facet model. A person's response, X_{pi}, to any item i can be broken down by,

$$X_{pi} = \mu + (\mu_p - \mu) + (\mu_i - \mu) + (X_{pi} - \mu_p - \mu_i + \mu), \tag{7}$$

where $\mu_p = \varepsilon X_{pi}$ = the row mean for person p in the matrix in Figure 1. This is the mean score for person p over *all* items in the universe of items;

$\mu_i = \underset{p}{\varepsilon} X_{pi}$ = the column mean for item i in the matrix in Figure 1. This is the mean score on item i over *all* persons in the population P; and

$\mu = \underset{p\,i}{\varepsilon\,\varepsilon} X_{pi}$ = the grand mean over all columns and rows in the matrix in Figure 1. This is the mean score over *all* items and over *all* persons.

The term μ_p is called person p's *universe score* and is the G-theory analog of Classical and IRT's true score.

A *Generalizability*, or *G-study* study would be conducted to characterize the universe of admissible observations represented by the matrix in Figure 1 and would lead to the variance breakdown,

$$\sigma^2(X_{pi}) = \sigma^2(p) + \sigma^2(i) + \sigma^2(pi,e), \qquad (8)$$

where $\sigma^2(X_{pi})$ = total variance of scores X_{pi},
$\sigma^2(p)$ = the variance of the row mean scores μ_p in the Figure 1 matrix;
$\sigma^2(i)$ = the variance of column mean scores μ_i in Figure 1;

and

$\sigma^2(pi,e)$ = variance of person-by-item interactions confounded with other sources of error.

A single facet measurement procedure based on this conceptualization would consist of a random sample of n_i' items from the universe of items being administered to a random sample of n_p' persons from the population.[3] Such a procedure would be characterized in a *Decision*, or *D-study*. Each person would have a mean score over the sample of n_i' items, X_{pI}, where the I subscript indicates the score is over a set of n_i' items. This mean score would be broken down in a manner analogous to equation (7):

$$X_{pI} = \mu + (\mu_p - \mu) + (\mu_I - \mu) + (X_{pI} - \mu_p - \mu_I + \mu), \qquad (9)$$

where μ_I = the population mean over the set of n_i' items. This decomposition is the Generalizability theory analog of Classical theory and Item Response Theory's decomposition of X into T + E. The score X_{pI} for person p would be used as an estimate of their universe score, μ_p.

Equation (9) would lead to the following variance breakdown:

$$\sigma^2(X_{pI}) = \sigma^2(p) + \sigma^2(I) + \sigma^2(pI,e), \qquad (10)$$

where $\sigma^2(I)$ = variance of distribution of all possible mean scores μ_I, where each mean μ_I is a mean for P over a different random sample of n_i' items.

FIGURE 1. Illustration of a Single Facet Generalizability Theory Model

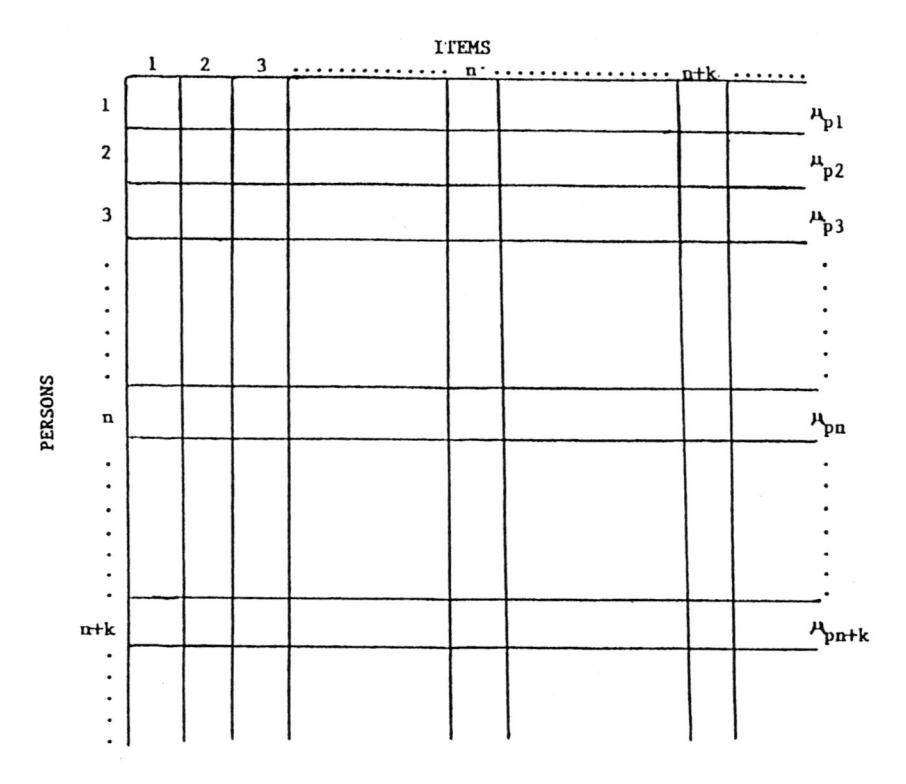

	ITEMS							
	1	2	3	.....	n·	.....	n+k	....
1								μ_{p1}
2								μ_{p2}
3								μ_{p3}
n								μ_{pn}
n+k								μ_{pn+k}

PERSONS

In this single facet model, $\sigma^2(p)$ is the variance of the universe scores μ_p, and is the Generalizability theory analog of Classical Theory's true score variance. The term $\sigma^2(pI,e)$ in equation (10) is identical to the error variance in Classical theory.

In Classical theory the assumption of parallel measures is equivalent to assuming that $\mu_I = \mu$ in equation (9), and, thus, that $\sigma^2(I) = 0$ in equation (10) (Brennan, 1983). Under this assumption, equation (10) reduces to,

$$\sigma^2(X_{pI}) = \sigma^2(p) + \sigma^2(pI,e). \tag{11}$$

This equation is equivalent to the Classical Theory decomposition

$$\sigma^2(X) = \sigma^2(T) + \sigma^2(E).$$

The assumption that $\sigma^2(I) = 0$ is the condition under which in a single facet model Generalizability Theory and Classical theory are essentially the same. Classical theory is not able to handle the case in which $\sigma^2(I) \neq 0$ (Brennan, 1983).

The simplest multifacet model is a two facet model. For example, consider the item-by-occasion matrix for person p shown in Figure 2A. This infinite matrix contains person p's responses to each of an infinite number of items on each of an infinite number of occasions. Each person would have such a matrix and combining these matrices for multiple persons to form a box, as shown in Figure 2B, creates a representation of the responses of all persons under all conditions in the universe of admissible observations for this two facet model.

A number of measurement procedures could be based on this universe of admissible observations. For example, each person in a random sample of size n_p' from P might respond to each of a random sample of n_i' items from the universe of items on each of a random sample of n_o' occasions from the universe of occasions. A person p's mean score over both n_i' items and n_o' occasions, X_{pIO}, would be used as an estimate of their universe score μ_p, where

$$\mu_p = \underset{o}{\varepsilon}\,\underset{i}{\varepsilon}\, X_{pio} = \text{the grand mean score over items and occasions in person p's item-by-occasion matrix shown in Figure 2A.}$$

The score X_{pIO} would have a breakdown that is a multifacet generalization of equation (9), and a variance decomposition that is a multifacet generalization of equation (10),

$$\sigma^2(X_{pIO}) = \sigma^2(p) + \sigma^2(I) + \sigma^2(O) + \sigma^2(pI) + \sigma^2(pO) + \sigma^2(IO) + \sigma^2(pIO,e). \tag{12}$$

RELIABILITY

The *Standards for Educational and Psychological Tests* (American Psychological Association, 1985) defines reliability as the "... degree to which test scores are free from errors of measurement." (p. 19). Both Item Response Theory and Generalizability Theory elaborate the theory of measurement error embodied in Classical Theory.

Classical Theory

In Classical Theory, reliability is defined as the squared correlation between observed scores and true scores, or equivalently, the ratio of true score variance to observed score variance:

$$\rho^2_{XT} = \sigma^2(T) \big/ \sigma^2(X), \tag{13}$$

where ρ^2_{XT} = squared correlation between observed and true scores.

FIGURE 2. Illustration of a Two Facet Generalizability Theory Model

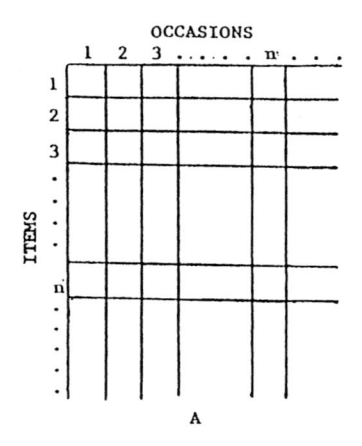

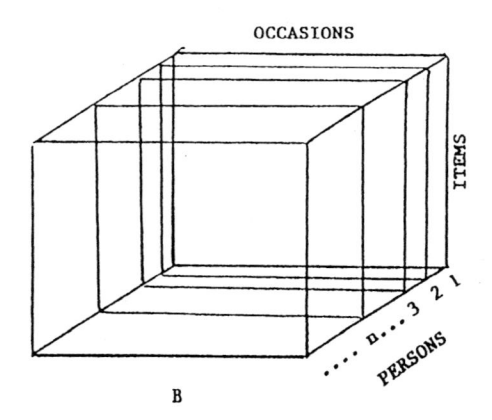

Reliability is estimated as the correlation between *strictly* parallel measurements (r_{xx}). The standard error of measurement (SEM) is the standard deviation of errors of measurement (Lord & Novick, 1968). The average SEM over a sample of persons is estimated by,

$$SEM = s_x \sqrt{1-r_{xx}} \qquad (14)$$

where: r_{xx} = the estimated reliability of the instrument, and

s_x = the standard deviation of observed scores on the instrument.

A crucial limitation of these Classical indices is that they are sample dependent. The estimated reliability, for example, can change from sample to sample within the same population (Hambleton & Swamanathan, 1985).

Item Response Theory

The score information function, $I(\theta,y)$ for any score y is defined as the square of the ratio of the slope of the regression of y on θ to the standard error of measurement for a given θ level (Hambleton & Swamanathan, 1985; Lord, 1980):

$$I(\theta,y) = \left[\frac{d}{d\theta}\varepsilon(y|\theta)\right]^2 \Big/ [\alpha(y|\theta)]^2 \qquad (15)$$

The square of the standard error of measurement at a given θ level, $\theta = \theta_0$, is given by the variance of y at θ_0. If the simple sum of responses to the items on a measurement instrument is used to estimate θ levels, the squared conditional standard error of measurement, according to Lord (1980), is given by:

$$\sigma^2(y|\theta_0) = \sum_{g=1}^{n} p_g(\theta) q_g(\theta) \qquad (16)$$

where $q_g(\theta) = 1 - p_g(\theta)$.
The squared standard error of measurement, SEM^2, of Classical theory is given by equation (16) averaged over all N persons responding to the instrument (Lord, 1980).

The *item information function* for the response u_g to item g, when the item response is modelled using the 2PL IRF, is produced by substituting equation (4) for $\varepsilon(y|\theta)$ in equation (15), giving,

$$I\left(\theta,\mu_g\right) = \frac{\left[1.7a_g\right]^2}{e^{1.7a_g(\theta-b_g)}\left[1 + e^{-1.7a_g(\theta-b_g)}\right]^2} \qquad (17)$$

where a_g = item g's *a* value, and b_g = item g's *b* value.
A graphic plot of an item's information at different θ levels is called the *item information curve* for the item (see Figure 5 in the sequel).

Imagine a four item depression scale which produces for each person a vector of item responses of the form $<u_1, u_2, u_3, u_4>$, where u_g represents the person's response to item g. In IRT, this vector of responses can be used in two ways to estimate the person's depression (i.e., θ) level. Maximum likelihood procedures may be applied to the untransformed vector to estimate the θ level most likely to lead to the observed vector for that person. When this procedure is used to estimate θ levels the information contribution by each item on the instrument to the total information given by the instrument is additive. The *test information function*, $I(\theta)$, which describes the precision in using the raw response vector to estimate θ levels, is given by the simple sum of all item information functions for the n items on the instrument:

$$I(\theta) = \sum_{g=1}^{n} I\{\theta, u_g\} . \qquad (18)$$

The test information function gives the maximum amount of information obtainable by *any* scoring procedure used with the n items (Lord, 1980). A graphic plot of the test information function [equation (18)] is called the *test information curve* (TIC). The height of the TIC is inversely related to the error associated with θ estimates at a given θ level:

$$SEE = 1/\sqrt{I(\theta)} \qquad (19)$$

where   SEE = standard error of estimated trait levels at a given θ level; the expected standard deviation of errors of estimated ability at a given level,
and $I(\theta)$ = amount of information (i.e., height of TIC) at the given θ level.

The average SEE ($\overline{SEE}$) is related to the classical reliability co-efficient when θ is scaled to a mean of 0 and a standard deviation of 1.0 (Warm, 1978):

$$r_{xx} = 1 - \overline{SEE}^2 . \qquad (20)$$

Both the SEE and r_{xx} are related to the nonlinear correlation, eta, between θ and the observed score X (Crocker & Algina, 1986):

$$eta = \sqrt{r_{xx}} = \sqrt{1 - \overline{SEE}^2} . \qquad (21)$$

The relationship in equation (20) and the continuous nature of the information function imply that an instrument with high reliability may be poor for some purposes because it has low information at critical θ levels. An instrument with low reliability, on the other hand, may be excellent for some purposes if it gives high information where needed. Thus, from an IRT perspective, Classical reliability estimates can be highly misleading as to the value of a measurement instrument (Warm, 1978).

The second way in which the vector $<u_1, u_2, u_3, u_4>$ may be used to estimate levels is to use some weighted or unweighted linear combination of the item responses to create a numerical score, such as the simple sum of item responses, $\sum_{g=1}^{4} u_g$. Unless some optimal item weighting procedure is used, however, the use of a linear combination of item responses to estimate θ levels will result is greater measurement error than will applying maximum likelihood procedures to the untransformed response vector (Warm, 1978; Lord, 1980).

Generalizability Theory

In G-theory the researcher uses an observed score, such as X_{pI} in a single facet design, as an estimate of a universe score, such as μ_p. In doing this the researcher is generalizing over a universe of measurements called the *universe of generalization*. For example, in the single facet model in which the facet is an item facet the universe of generalization is over all items in the universe of items. That is, the researcher wants to generalize from X_{pI} to the row mean $\mu_p = \varepsilon X_{pi}$ in the person-by-item matrix of Figure 1. The theory of measurement error within G-theory focuses upon the errors involved in using an observed score as an estimate of a universe score (Cronbach et al., 1972; Brennan, 1983).

In a single facet design the *relative error variance*, $\sigma^2(\delta)$, is given by,

$$\sigma^2(\delta) = \sigma^2(pI,e) . \tag{22}$$

This is the variance of the error δ, defined as,

$$\delta = (X_{pI} - \mu_I) - (\mu_p - \mu) . \tag{23}$$

This is the error involved in using a person's observed deviation score, $X_{pI} - X_{PI}$ (where X_{PI} = observed mean over persons and items), as an estimate of their universe deviation score, $\mu_p - \mu$ (Cronbach et al., 1972). This is the error variance of concern whenever the researcher wishes to make relative comparisons of scores (Brennan, 1983). As noted earlier, in a single facet design the D-study variance component $\sigma^2(pI,e)$ is equivalent to the Classical error variance. Thus, $\sigma^2(\delta)$ in the single facet model is the same as the Classical error variance, regardless of whether or not $\sigma^2(I) = 0$ (Brennan, 1983). This is because the definition of δ is such that μ_I is a constant for all persons in the deviation scores of interest. Thus, even though $\sigma^2(I)$ may not be 0, it does not contribute to $\sigma^2(\delta)$.

In the single facet model the *absolute error variance*, $\sigma^2(\Delta)$, is given by,

$$\sigma^2(\Delta) = \sigma^2(I) + \sigma^2(pI,e) = \sigma^2(I) + \sigma^2(\delta). \tag{24}$$

This is the variance of the error Δ, defined as,

$$\Delta = X_{pI} - \mu_p. \tag{25}$$

This is the error involved in using a person's observed score X_{pI} as an estimate of their universe score, μ_p (Brennan, 1983). Error variance $\sigma^2(\Delta)$ is of concern anytime the researcher wishes to make absolute decisions regarding a person, such as what her/his universe score might be or how the person's universe score compares with a set standard (Brennan, 1983).

It can be seen from equations (22) and (24) that,

$$\sigma^2(\Delta) \geq \sigma^2(\delta), \tag{26}$$

with equality holding only if $\sigma^2(I) = 0$. Thus, Classical theory, since it assumes that $\sigma^2(I) = 0$, cannot make the distinction between $\sigma^2(\delta)$ and $\sigma^2(\Delta)$. As a result of the assumption of parallel measures, $\sigma^2(\delta) = \sigma^2(\Delta)$ in Classical theory. One consequence of this is that in the single facet design a confidence interval for a true (universe) score formed using Classical methods will generally be smaller than that formed using G-theory methods. This is because $\sigma^2(\Delta)$ is the appropriate error variance to use in forming such a confidence interval and unless $\sigma^2(I) = 0$,

$$\sigma(\Delta) > \sigma(\delta) = \text{SEM}. \tag{27}$$

The *generalizability coefficient*, $\varepsilon\rho^2$, is defined as,

$$\varepsilon\rho^2 = \frac{\sigma^2(p)}{\sigma^2(p) + \sigma^2(\delta)} = \frac{\text{universe score variance}}{\text{expected observed score variance}}. \tag{28}$$

This is the ratio of universe score variance to expected observed score variance; it is also the expected squared correlation between observed and universe scores (Brennan, 1983). An equivalent interpretation is that it is the expected correlation between observed scores on two randomly parallel instances of the measurement procedure. For the single facet case, with items the facet of interest, a randomly parallel instance of the measurement procedure will be a different random sample of n_i' items (Cronbach et al., 1972; Brennan, 1983). For the single facet model the generalizability coefficient is given by,

$$\varepsilon\rho^2 = \frac{\sigma^2(p)}{\sigma^2(p) + \sigma^2(pI,e)}. \tag{29}$$

If the same number of items are used in a single facet D-study as in the G-study of the universe of admissible observations, then $\varepsilon\rho^2$ will be numerically equal to the Classically based reliability estimate coefficient alpha. This correspondence does not, however, in general apply when the researcher wishes to generalize over more than one facet. There will be at least three different universe scores for the item and occasion two facet model discussed earlier. The first would be $\mu_p = \underset{O}{\varepsilon}\underset{I}{\varepsilon} X_{pIo}$, the grand mean score in the item-by-occasion matrix for person p shown in Figure 2A. This is the grand mean over all items in the universe of items and over all occasions in the universe of occasions. The relative error variance for this universe of generalization is given by,

$$\sigma^2(\delta) = \sigma^2(pI) + \sigma^2(pO) + \sigma^2(pIO,e) . \tag{30}$$

The absolute error variance is given by,

$$\sigma^2(\Delta) = \sigma^2(I) + \sigma^2(O) + \sigma^2(pI) + \sigma^2(pO) \\ + \sigma^2(IO) + \sigma^2(pIO,e) . \tag{31}$$

The generalizability coefficient will be given by equation (28) with equation (30) substituted for the term $\sigma^2(\delta)$.

A second universe score to which the researcher may wish to generalize in this two facet model is the person's mean score over *only* the n_i' items used in the measurement procedure *and* over all occasions in the universe of occasions: $\mu_{pi^*} = \underset{O}{\varepsilon} X_{pI^*o}$, where I^* indicates the set of n_i' items in the measurement procedure. This universe of generalization is illustrated in Figure 3A. In this Figure the item-by-occasion matrix for person p is shown with a subregion of the matrix crosshatched. The mean score μ_{pi^*} is the grand mean over the crosshatched area in Figure 3A. The relative error variance for this *restricted universe of generalization* is given by,

$$\sigma^2(\delta) = \sigma^2(pO) + \sigma^2(pIO,e) , \tag{32}$$

while the absolute error variance is given by,

$$\sigma^2(\Delta) = \sigma^2(O) + \sigma^2(pO) + \sigma^2(IO) + \sigma^2(pIO,e) . \tag{33}$$

The generalizability coefficient is given by,

$$\varepsilon\rho^2 = \frac{\sigma^2(p) + \sigma^2(pI)}{\sigma^2(p) + \sigma^2(pI) + \sigma^2(\delta)} , \tag{34}$$

with equation (32) substituted for the term $\sigma^2(\delta)$. The reader will note that the error variances for the restricted universe of generalization are smaller, the universe score variance larger $[\sigma^2(p) + \sigma^2(pI)]$, and the generalizability coefficient larger than the corresponding indices for the unrestricted universe of generalization. A third possible universe of generalization is represented by the crosshatched area in Figure 3B. This would be generalizing over all items in the universe of items and over only the n'_o occasions in the measurement procedure.

AN APPLIED COMPARATIVE ANALYSIS

Three-hundred-forty responses were obtained on the Generalized Contentment Scale (GCS) (Hudson, 1982) from university students and outpatients receiving psychotherapy in a community mental health center. The GCS measures depression using 25 items with item responses ranging from 1 ("Rarely or none of the time") to 5 ("Most or all of the time"). To facilitate an IRT analysis, the item responses on the GCS were dichotomized, with items originally scored 1 rescored to 0, and items with original scores of 2 or above rescored to 1. The logic behind this rescoring is that if an item was originally scored a 1, then the characteristic described by the item was most likely *not true* for the respondent. Similarly, any item originally scored 2 or higher described a characteristic that likely was *true* for the respondent. These dichotomized responses were analyzed using Classical and IRT procedures.[4] A second sample of responses on the GCS was obtained and analyzed using G-theory methods. This second sample is described in more detail below.

The dichotomized GCS data were Classically analyzed using the Reliability subprogram of SPSS (Nie, Hull, Jenkins, Steinbrenner, and Bent, 1975). The coefficient alpha estimate of reliability for this set of responses is .91. Thus, the estimated correlation between true and observed scores is $\sqrt{.91}$ = .954. The estimated SEM for these data is 1.96. The non-dichotomized GCS data were also analyzed using SPSS Reliability. The coefficient alpha estimate of reliability for this polytomous data is .938, with a SEM of 4.2. These latter results compare well with those given by Hudson (1982).

A 2PL IRF model was fitted to the dichotomized GCS data using the program LOGIST IV (Wingersky, Barton, and Lord, 1982).[5] Table 1 shows the estimated item parameters for the 2PL IRF model for the 25 dichotomized GCS items.

Figure 4 shows the ICCs for dichotomized items 4 and 9. The reader will note the differing slopes of these ICCs. The maximum slope of item 4 is much less than the maximum slope of item 9. This indicates that item 9 does a better job of discriminating between levels of depression than does item 4. The reader will also note the differing locations along the θ continuum, shown on the horizontal axis, that the maximum slope of these ICCs covers. The locations along the θ scale that the maximum slopes of the ICCs cover indicate the differing ranges along the θ continuum at which the items function to discriminate maximally between different levels of θ.

FIGURE 3. Illustration of Restricted Universes of Generalization in a Two Facet Generalizability Theory Model

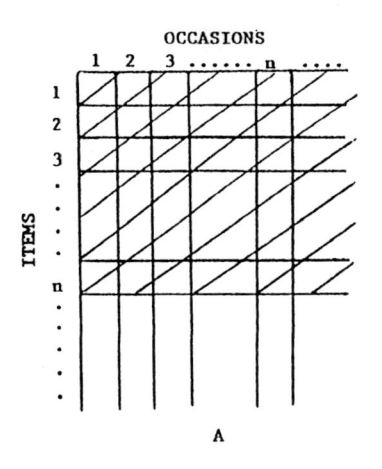

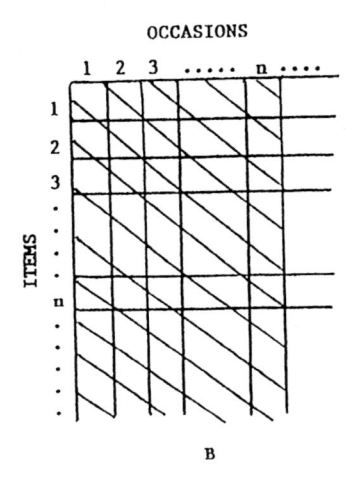

Table 1: Item Parameter Estimates for 2PL IRF Model Fitted to Dichotomized GCS Data

Item	Estimated a value	Estimated b value
1	1.106	-0.163
2	1.016	-1.041
3	0.402	-0.981
4	0.513	0.947
5	0.595	-1.724
6	0.473	-2.245
7	0.547	-0.239
8	0.914	-0.176
9	2.000	-0.316
10	1.770	-0.418
11	1.089	-0.478
12	1.152	-0.829
13	0.724	0.082
14	0.973	0.801
15	0.790	-0.295
16	0.968	-0.901
17	1.928	-0.037
18	0.493	-1.635
19	0.830	-0.998
20	1.243	-0.134
21	1.566	-0.282
22	1.029	-0.219
23	1.530	-0.905
24	0.961	-1.377
25	1.375	0.704

a values: mean = 1.0395   sd = .4435329
b values: mean = -.5144   sd = .7541837

Figure 5 shows the item information functions for items 4 and 9. In this figure the height of an item's information curve at a given θ level indicates the information provided by the item for distinguishing between different trait levels. The differing heights of the two item information functions at different θ levels shows that each item provides different amounts of information at these θ levels. At θ levels where its information curve is higher, item 4 gives more information about the level of depression than does item 9. However, at θ levels where its information curve is higher, item 9 gives more information than does item 4. The reader will also note the difference in the maximum height of the two item information functions. The maximum information value for item 9 (about 2.8) is about 15 times larger than the maximum for item 4 (about .19). This is due

FIGURE 4. Item Characteristic Curves for Dichotomized Items Number 4 and 9 on Hudson's Generalized Contentment Scale

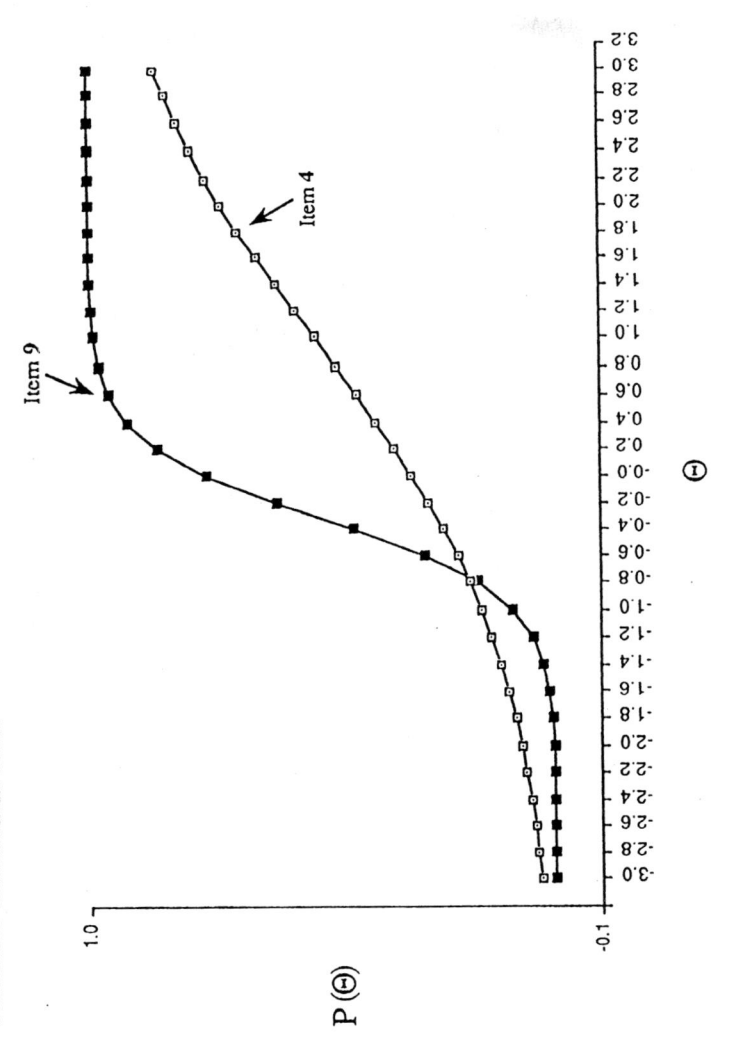

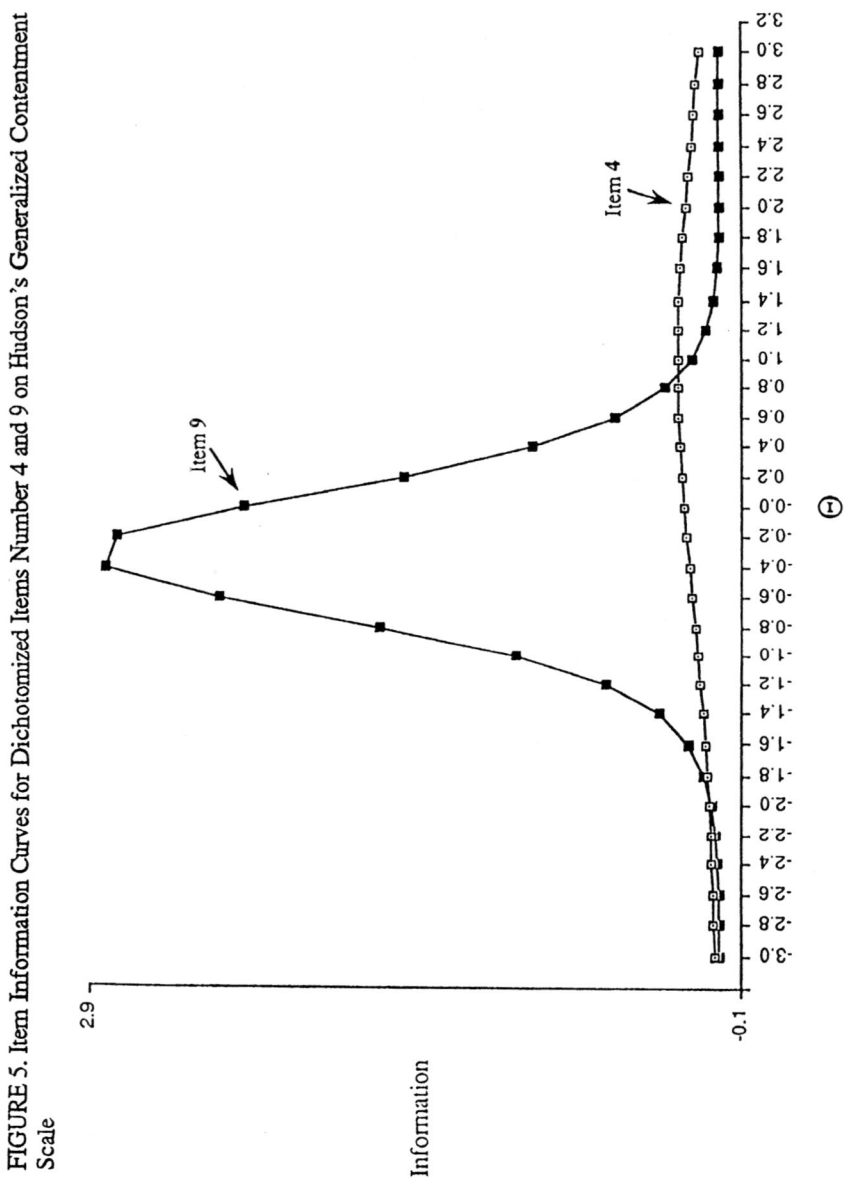

FIGURE 5. Item Information Curves for Dichotomized Items Number 4 and 9 on Hudson's Generalized Contentment Scale

primarily to the difference in the *a* parameter values for these two items (a = 2.0 for item 9; a = .513 for item 4). The value of the *a* parameter is a major determinant of the amount of information given by an item in the 2PL IRF model [see equation (17)], with larger *a* values for items leading to greater amounts of information (Hambleton & Swamanathan, 1985).

Figure 6 shows the TIC for the dichotomized version of the GCS. As will be remembered from earlier discussion, this curve gives the *maximum* amount of information about θ levels obtainable by any scoring procedure used with the 25 GCS dichotomized items. Since a 2PL IRF model was fitted to the GCS dichotomized data, this curve also gives the information provided about θ levels by the weighted sum, X_w, of GCS item responses given by,

$$X_w = \sum_{g=1}^{25} a_g u_g \qquad (35)$$

where a_g = the *a* value for item g, and u_g = response on item g. This is one of the advantages of using a 2PL IRF model; the *a* values for each item are the optimal item weights to use in computing a weighted sum of item scores for use in estimating θ levels (Lord & Novick, 1968; Lord, 1980). Any other scoring procedure, such as the simple sum of item responses, will give less information than either the scoring procedure in equation (35) or maximum likelihood estimates based on the vector of item responses as described earlier.

Table 2 gives the measurement error characteristics of the dichotomized GCS. The reader will note that the lowest standard error of estimate values are associated with the *largest* standard error of measurement values, and vice versa. Lord and Novick (1968) discuss this paradox, which can partly be understood as follows. Equation (5) describes the functional relationship between true score, T, and θ. This relationship, shown graphically in Figure 7, is nonlinear and is called the *test characteristic curve*. The reader will note that very high and very low dichotomized GCS true scores functionally relate to the θ metric in regions where the slope of the test characteristic curve is very low. Thus, large ranges of θ values, which have an unlimited range, are squeezed into very small ranges of GCS true scores. This compression of large θ ranges into small true score ranges explains, in part, the paradoxical relationship between the standard error of estimate and the standard error of measurement seen in Table 2. This result highlights some of the limitations in the Classical theory concept of the standard error of measurement (Samejima, 1977; Hambleton & Swamanathan, 1985). The reader can compare the results shown in Table 2 with the Classical SEM estimate of 1.96 for the dichotomized GCS.

In a second sample, one-hundred-ten responses were obtained on the GCS, fifty-five on each of two occasions one-week apart, from outpatient psychotherapy clients. These responses were dichotomized and then both dichotomized and non-dichotomized data were analyzed in a two-facet Generalizability analysis

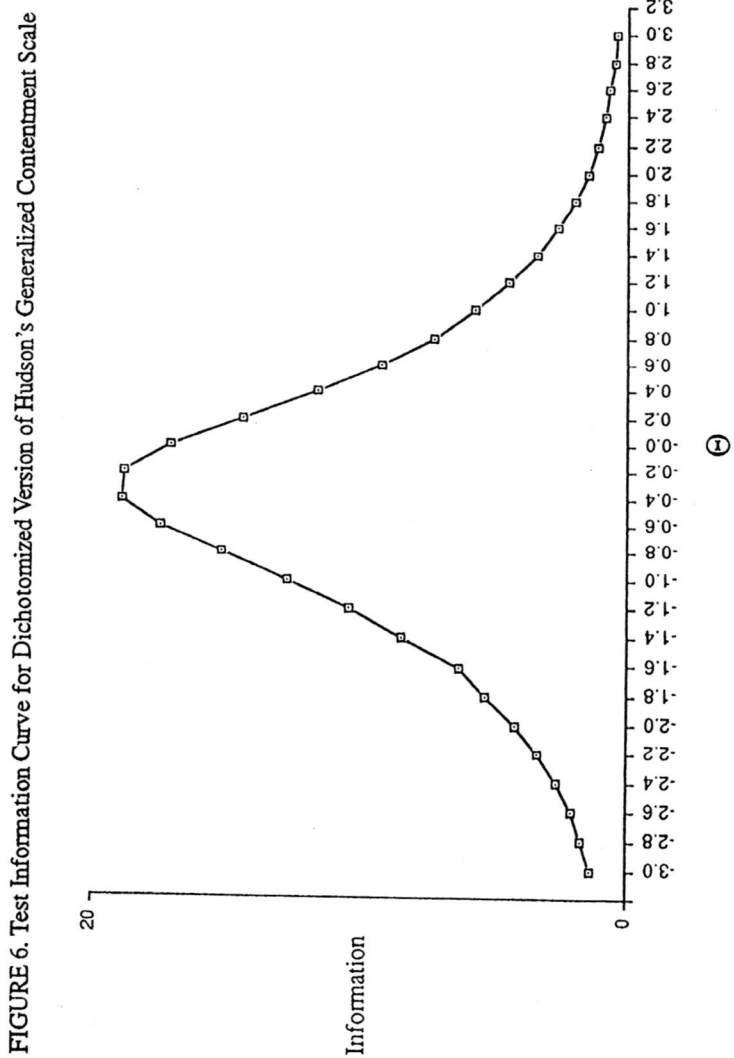

FIGURE 6. Test Information Curve for Dichotomized Version of Hudson's Generalized Contentment Scale

Table 2: Measurement Error Characteristics of Dichotomized GCS

θ Level	Information	Standard Error of θ Estimate	Standard Error of Measurement in Total Score Metric
-3.0	1.337	.86484	1.057
-2.8	1.663	.77545	1.134
-2.6	2.082	.69304	1.218
-2.4	2.620	.61780	1.309
-2.2	3.312	.54948	1.406
-2.0	4.198	.48807	1.511
-1.8	5.323	.43343	1.622
-1.6	6.730	.38547	1.738
-1.4	8.451	.34399	1.855
-1.2	10.489	.30877	1.968
-1.0	12.801	.27950	2.073
-0.8	15.264	.25596	2.162
-0.6	17.541	.23877	2.227
-0.4	18.973	.22958	2.253
-0.2	18.873	.23019	2.228
0.0	17.157	.24142	2.151
0.2	14.476	.26283	2.037
0.4	11.670	.29273	1.906
0.6	9.243	.32892	1.772
0.8	7.288	.37042	1.640
1.0	5.717	.41823	1.510
1.2	4.441	.47453	1.384
1.4	3.413	.54129	1.263
1.6	2.602	.61993	1.149
1.8	1.976	.71139	1.044
2.0	1.501	.81622	0.949
2.2	1.144	.93495	0.864
2.4	0.878	1.06722	0.787
2.6	0.680	1.21268	0.717
2.8	0.528	1.37620	0.655
3.0	0.414	1.55417	0.599

using BMDP08V (Dixon & Brown, 1979). Two D-studies were performed, one for each of two possible universes of generalization: (1) for generalizing over all items in the universe of items and over all occasions in the universe of occasions (i.e., over both facets), and (2) for generalizing over only the 25 GCS items and over all occasions in the universe of occasions. The results of the analysis of the non-dichotomized data are shown in the first two columns of Table 3, while the results of the analysis of the dichotomized data are shown in the first two columns of the lower portion of Table 4.

As can be seen in these tables, the error variances and generalizability coefficients differ for each universe of generalization. The error variances are smaller, and the generalizability coefficients larger, for the restricted universe of generalization. These are the effects of fixing a facet as a means of standardizing a measurement procedure (Cronbach et al., 1982). However, the price paid for

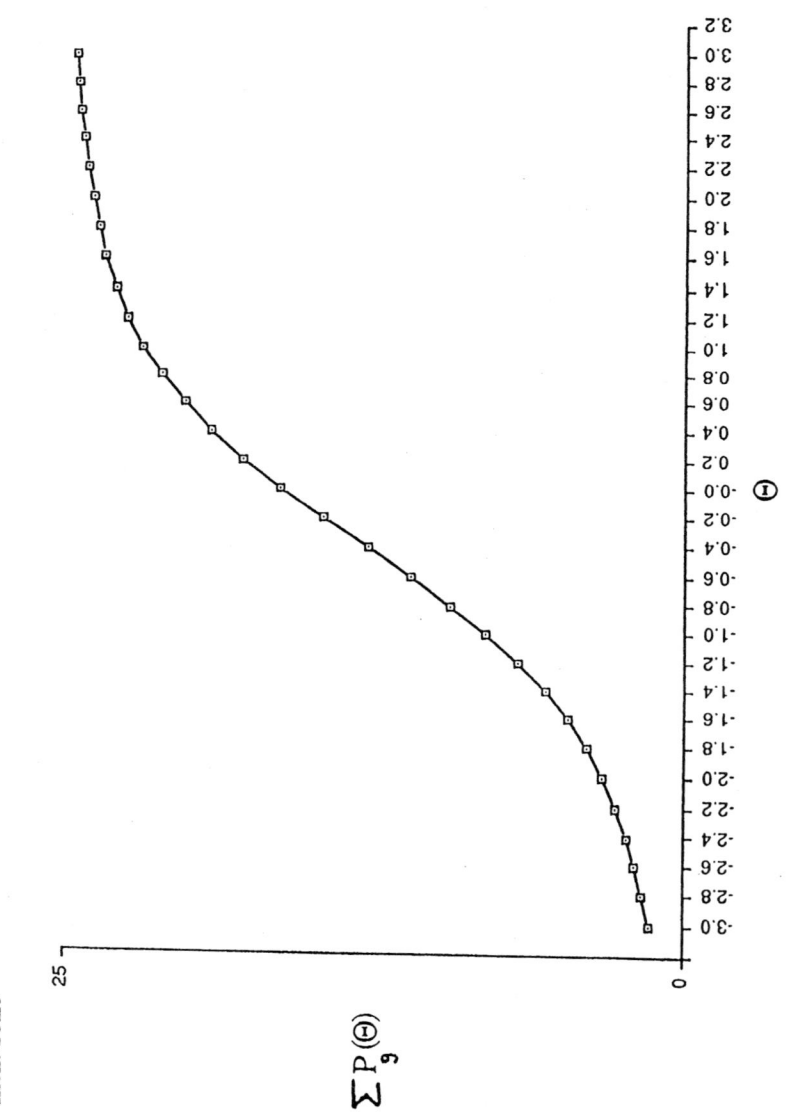

FIGURE 7. Test Characteristic Curve Relating True Score and θ Metrics on Dichotomized Generalized Content-ment Scale

this is a more limited scope of generalization and, quite possibly, a decrease in validity (Kane, 1982).

A useful comparison between Classical and G-theory conceptualizations of a measurement procedure can be made by considering the commonly used approach to estimating the Classical reliability of an instrument, such as the GCS, in which the scale is administered to a sample of subjects on a single occasion and then coefficient alpha computed. As discussed earlier, in G-theory terms this is essentially a single facet D-study design with the universe of generalization being over the item facet (Brennan, 1983). In this universe of generalization, the occasion of administration is kept fixed at $n_o' = 1$; that is, there is an occasion facet in which the number of occasions in the universe of occasions, N_o', is unity: $N_o' = 1$. In this situation, the occasion facet is said to be "hidden"; that is, it is not explicitly considered in the research design but is implicit. The third column in Table 3, and the third column in the lower portion of Table 4, gives the D-study results for a single facet D-study design in which

Table 3: Results of G-theory Analysis of Non-Dichotomized GCS Data

Results in Total Score Metric

Results with $n_o'=2$ and $n_i'=25$, and for generalizing over both item and occasion facets	Results with n_i' fixed at 25, $n_o'=2$, and for generalizing over $n_i'=25$ items and occasion facet	Results with $n_o'=N_o'=1$, $n_i'=25$, and for generalizing over both facets	Results with $n_o'=1$, $n_i'=25$, and for generalizing over both item and occasion facets
$\sigma^2(\delta) = 20.75$	$\sigma^2(\delta) = 12.33$	$\sigma^2(\delta) = 17.89$	$\sigma^2(\delta) = 33.09$
$\sigma(\delta) = 4.555$	$\sigma(\delta) = 3.511$	$\sigma(\delta) = 4.229$	$\sigma(\delta) = 5.7522$
$\sigma^2(\Delta) = 24.97$	$\sigma^2(\Delta) = 14.02$	$\sigma^2(\Delta) = 20.41$	$\sigma^2(\Delta) = 38.99$
$\sigma(\Delta) = 4.997$	$\sigma(\Delta) = 3.744$	$\sigma(\Delta) = 4.518$	$\sigma(\Delta) = 6.244$
$\varepsilon\rho^2 = .941$	$\varepsilon\rho^2 = .965$	$\varepsilon\rho^2 = .951$	$\varepsilon\rho^2 = .909$
95% CI: X ± 9.8	95% CI: X ± 7.3	95% CI: X ± 8.3	95% CI: X ± 12.2

Table 4: Comparative Results of Classical, IRT, and G-theory Analyses of Dichotomized GCS Data

Classical	IRT
SCALE	SCALE
$r_{xx} = .91$	$I\{\theta,y\}$: varies with θ according to equation (15); see Figure 6.
SEM = 1.96	SEM: varies with θ according to equation (16); see Table 2.
95% Confidence Interval: $X \pm 3.84$	SEE: varies with θ according to equation (19); see Table 2.
ITEMS	ITEMS
item 4:	item 4:
p = .358	$p(\theta)$: varies with θ according to equation (4); see Figure 4.
corrected item-total correlation = .37	$I\{\theta,u\}$: varies with θ according to equation (17); see Figure 5.
item 9:	item 9:
p = .60	$p(\theta)$: varies with θ according to equation (4); see Figure 4.
corrected item-total correlation = .70	$I\{\theta,u\}$: varies with θ according to equation (17); see Figure 5.

G-theory (results in total score metric)

Results with $n_o'=2$ and $n_i'=25$, and for generalizing over both item and occasion facets	Results with n_i' fixed at 25, $n_o'=2$, and for generalizing over $n_i'=25$ items and occasion facet	Results with $n_o'=N_o'=1$, $n_i'=25$, and for generalizing over both facets	Results with $n_o'=1$, $n_i'=25$, and for generalizing over both item and occasion facets
$\sigma^2(\delta) = 3.227$	$\sigma^2(\delta) = 1.763$	$\sigma^2(\delta) = 2.915$	$\sigma^2(\delta) = 4.991$
$\sigma(\delta) = 1.797$	$\sigma(\delta) = 1.328$	$\sigma(\delta) = 1.707$	$\sigma(\delta) = 2.2342$
$\sigma^2(\Delta) = 3.602$	$\sigma^2(\Delta) = 1.826$	$\sigma^2(\Delta) = 3.234$	$\sigma^2(\Delta) = 5.428$
$\sigma(\Delta) = 1.898$	$\sigma(\Delta) = 1.351$	$\sigma(\Delta) = 1.798$	$\sigma(\Delta) = 2.32$
$\varepsilon\rho^2 = .896$	$\varepsilon\rho^2 = .943$	$\varepsilon\rho^2 = .911$	$\varepsilon\rho^2 = .847$
95% CI: $X \pm 3.7$	95% CI: $X \pm 2.7$	95% CI: $X \pm 3.6$	95% CI: $X \pm 4.6$

the occasion facet is hidden (i.e., where $n_o' = 1$, and $N_o' = 1$). This is essentially a study equivalent to the type generally done to estimate the reliability of an instrument using Classical methods (Brennan, 1983). In this case the intended generalization is over a universe containing an infinite number of items administered only on a single occasion. The fourth column in Table 3, and the fourth column in the lower portion of Table 4, give the D-study results for a two facet design in which only a single occasion is sampled from the infinite universe of occasions (i.e., $n_o' = 1$, and $N_o' \to \infty$). In this latter case, the intended generalization is across a universe containing an infinite number of items administered on an infinite number of occasions (i.e., over both facets).

If the researcher is willing to grant that the occasion of administration of an instrument may contain influences that lead to error in GCS responses, then the investigator will want to generalize over a universe containing an infinite number of occasions as opposed to a universe of generalization which contains a single occasion. Thus the occasion facet contains more than a single occasion, whether or not the researcher has explicitly considered the occasion facet as a source of error in the reliability study. However, the generalizability coefficients shown in the third column of Table 3 (.951) and the third column of the lower portion of Table 4 (.911) are the figures likely to be obtained as reliability estimates in the classical one-time administration of the GCS. The generalizability coefficient in the fourth columns (.909 and .847, respectively) are more indicative of the reliabilities when the hidden occasion facet is explicitly considered. As can be seen, the reliability estimates will be lower when the hidden facet is considered. As Brennan (1983) notes, the results in the fourth columns may be more in line with the types of generalizations that most investigators would like to make when all items are administered on the same occasion.

> ... if one wants to generalize over occasions, then an internal consistency coefficient is likely to be an over-estimate, and the classical error variance is likely to be an underestimate. (p. 86)

SUMMARY

Table 4 contains a comparison of results from Classical, IRT, and G-theory analyses of the dichotomized GCS data. Results for the entire scale and for items 4 and 9 are shown. As can be seen, the Classical and G-theory results are point estimates of performance indices. In contrast, the IRT results are continuous functions of the characteristic measured by the items on the instrument.

The Classical coefficient alpha estimate of reliability is 0.91, a figure essentially identical to the G-theory estimate of $\varepsilon\rho^2$ for the hidden facet case (i.e., where $n_o' = N_o' = 1$). The values for $\varepsilon\rho^2$ differ, however, from the Classical reliability estimate for different universes of generalization. The Classical estimate of the SEM (based on n = 340 sample) is 1.96, while the G-theory estimate of $\sigma(\delta)$ in the hidden facet case is 1.71 (based on n = 55 and two occasion sample).[6] IRT, in contrast, does not produce a single number reliability estimate. Instead, the functions $I\{\theta,y\}$, $\sigma^2(y|\theta)$, and SEE provide descriptions of measurement precision across the range of levels of the trait being measured. The IRT estimate of SEM ranges from 0.599 to 2.25, depending upon the level of the respondent.

The different G-theory results for the error terms $\sigma(\delta)$ and $\sigma(\Delta)$, as well as for the generalizability coefficients, for the different universes of generalization give an indication of the extent to which measurement error descriptors can vary depending upon the generalizations the researcher wishes to make. The results for the non-dichotomized data in Table 3 also show the variability in standard error estimates and generalizability coefficients depending upon the universe of generalization desired by the researcher. This variability underscores the importance of the researcher carefully determining the desired universe of generalization for a given measurement application.

Another useful comparison can be made between Classical theory and G-theory by considering the 95% confidence intervals for a person's universe, or true, score. Hudson (1982) reports a clinical cutting score of 30 on the GCS.[7] Scores of 30 or higher are evidence of a clinically significant problem with depression. A 95% confidence interval for a person's true score when her/his observed score is 30 would be, using Classical methods, 21.8 to 38.2. This interval is nearly identical to that obtained from G-theory methods when occasion is considered as a hidden facet: 21.7 to 38.3. In contrast, when occasion is explicitly considered as a facet, and the GCS is administered on only a single occasion the interval is 17.8 to 42.2. If the GCS is administered on two occasions, the interval shrinks to 20.2 to 39.8. If the item facet is fixed and generalization is desired over only the 25 items on the GCS and over the occasion facet, the interval shrinks further to 22.7 to 37.4. Confidence intervals are not usually formed in IRT.

Table 4 shows two Classical item performance indices: the item p-value (the proportion of respondents scoring the item 1) and the corrected item-total correlation. As with the Classical scale performance indices, these are point estimates. In contrast the IRT item performance descriptors $p(\theta)$ and $I\{\theta,u\}$ are continuous functions of θ. G-theory gives no indices of item performance. G-theory will view any item as merely one condition of the item facet and will provide variance components describing the variability in scores associated with different items being sampled from the universe of items.

VALIDITY

The validation of a measurement procedure developed within Classical, IRT, or Generalizability theories will involve essentially the same procedures. There are no differences in the conceptualization of instrument validation between these three theories. Indeed, validity can be viewed as a developing theory that stands essentially separate from Classical, IRT, and Generalizability theories.

CONCLUDING DISCUSSION

Suppose that research has shown that a depression level of $\theta = 1.2$ (a true score of about 22 on the dichotomized GCS) or greater identifies clients who are suicidal and that the researcher wishes to develop an instrument to use to classify persons as either suicidal or non-suicidal. Thus, an instrument that measures most reliably in the neighborhood of the true score of 22 is needed. The Classical p-values for items 4 and 9 are $p_4 = .358$ and $p_9 = .60$, while the corrected item-total correlations for items 4 and 9 are, respectively, .37 and .70. Given these indices, Classical theory would suggest that item 9 will function in a manner superior to item 4. However, the item information functions (see Figure 5) for these items leads to a different conclusion. The height of the item information curve for item 4 at $\theta = 1.2$ is approximately twice as high as that for item 9. For the purposes of the researcher, item 4 is actually superior to item 9. In a similar vein, the Classical reliability of .91 for this scale suggests good reliability characteristics. However, the test information curve (see Figure 6) shows that the instrument provides very little information at $\theta = 1.2$. Indeed, Table 2 shows the SEE at this θ level to be .47, a rather large error compared to the .229 at $\theta = -4$. Thus, the IRT results lead to different conclusions regarding the relative merit of items 4 and 9 and about the instrument as a whole than would the Classical results for this particular application.

In this application G-theory will tell the researcher little concerning the relative functioning of the two items. The D-study variance components will inform the researcher about the error introduced into measurements from the use of different sized samples of items from the universe of items. However, it will give the researcher nothing to help in terms of deciding which item performs better. If a multifacet G-study was conducted the variance components can be used to determine ways of minimizing the contribution to measurement error made by specific conditions of measurement, something that neither Classical theory nor IRT can do.

As another example, suppose that a researcher wishes to develop a measurement procedure to measure level of depression in which different persons are administered *different sets of items*. Further, suppose that the researcher wants to compare the scores over the different sets of items and make determinations as to relative severity of depression. Classical theory will be of no use to this researcher. Item Response Theory can be used in what is called adaptive testing to do this very thing (Crocker & Algina, 1986). G-theory methods could also be used in an application such as this. G-theory methods could be used to estimate error variances and generalizability coefficients for this measurement operation in which items are nested under persons (Brennan, 1983).

Numerous other examples could be given to demonstrate the different applications and capabilities of these theories. As the above examples and earlier discussion suggest, IRT and G-theory open the door to measurement and assessment technology not possible with Classical theory. The application and use of methods from these two theories can greatly broaden the research and development possibilities open to the social work researcher.

REFERENCE NOTES

1. Scores on the GCS can range from 0 to 100, with higher scores indicative of more severe depression. Hudson (1982) reports a coefficient alpha reliability estimate of .92 on a sample of 2140 respondents, with a standard error of measurement of 4.26.

2. Most current IRT models assume that items are scored dichotomously. The development in this paper is based upon this assumption. An IRT model for graded responses or polychotomously scored items was developed by Samejima (1969). However, it has not been until recently that computer software became available for this model and research and development on the graded response model is still in its early stages relative to the dichotomously scored models. Since the graded response model is built upon a dichotomously scored model, we have presented a model assuming dichotomously scored items.

3. In G-theory symbolism a lower-case n indicates a sample size in a G-study. An apostrophe (') by a lower-case n (n') indicates that the sample is being used in a D-study. This convention is used throughout the text of this article. Thus, for example, n_i would indicate that there are n items in a G-study, while n_i' would indicate the number of items from the universe of items that has been randomly selected for use in a D-study.

4. The GCS data were dichotomized to facilitate an IRT analysis. The dichotomized data were analyzed using procedures from all three theories in order to facilitate a comparison of results (see Table 4).

5. A copy of LOGIST IV can be obtained from Educational Testing Service, Princeton, New Jersey. Educational Testing Service owns the copyright on LOGIST software.

6. The reader will remember that in Classical theory the assumption is made that $\sigma^2(1) = 0$, and so $\sigma(\delta) = \sigma(\Delta)$. Thus, since the hidden facet case is essentially a single facet design, the term $\sigma(\delta)$ would be equivalent to the Classical SEM. In other G-theory designs described in this paper, the term $\sigma(\Delta)$ would be used to estimate the standard error associated with estimates of a person's universe (true) score.

7. This cut score is for the non-dichotomized GCS.

REFERENCES

Allen, M.J. & Yen, W.M. (1979). *Introduction to Measurement Theory*. Monterey, CA: Brooks/Cole.

American Psychological Association, American Educational Research Association, & National Council on Measurement in Education. (1985). *Standards* for *Educational and Psychological Testing*. Washington, D.C.: American Psychological Association.

Bloom, M., Fischer, J. (1982). *Evaluating Practice*. New Jersey: Prentice Hall.

Brennan, R. (1983). *Elements of Generalizability Theory*. Iowa City, Iowa: ACT Publications.

Corcoran, K., Fischer, J. (1987). *Measures for Clinical Practice*. New York: The Free Press.

Crocker, L., Algina, J. (1986). *Introduction to Classical & Modern Test Theory*. Chicago: Holt, Rinehart, and Winston.

Cronbach, L.J.; Gleser, G.C.; Nanda, H.; & Rajaratnam, N. (1972). *The Dependability of Behavioral Measurements: Theory of Generalizability for Scores and Profiles*. New York: Wiley.

Dixon, W., Brown, M. (Eds.) (1979). *BMDP-79 Biomedical Computer Programs, P. Series*. Los Angeles, California: University of California Press.

Ghiselli, E.E.; Campbell, J.P.; & Zedeck, S. (1981). *Measurement Theory for the Behavioral Sciences*. San Francisco: W.H. Freeman.

Hambleton, R.K. & Swaminathan, H. (1985). *Item Response Theory: Principles and Applications*. Boston: Kluwer-Nijhoff.

Hudson, W. (1982) *The Clinical Measurement Package*. Homewood, Ill.: Dorsey Press.

Kane, M. (1982). "A sampling model for validity." *Applied Psychological Measurement, 6*, 125-160.

Kerlinger, F. (1973). *Foundations of Behavioral Research*. New York: Holt, Rinehart, & Winston.

Lord, F.M. (1980). *Applications of Item Response Theory to Practical Testing Problems*. Hillsdale, NJ: Lawrence Erlbaum.

Lord, F.M. & Novick, M.R. (1968). *Statistical Theories of Mental Test Scores*. Reading, Mass.: Addison-Wesley.

Nie, N., Hull, C., Jenkins, J., Steinbrenner, K., and Bent, D. (1975). *Statistical Package for the Social Sciences* (2ed.). New York: McGraw-Hill.

Nunnally, J.C. (1978). *Psychometric Theory*. New York: McGraw-Hill.

Samejima, F. (1969). Estimation of latent ability using a response pattern of graded scores. *Psychometric Monograph*, No. 17.

Samejima, F. (1977). A use of the information function in tailored testing. *Applied Psychological Measurement. 1*, 233-247.

Shavelson, R., Webb, N., and Rowley, G. (1989). "Generalizability theory." *American Psychologist, 44*, 922-932.

Warm, T.A. (1978). *A Primer of Item Response Theory*. Oklahoma City, OK: U.S. Coast Guard Institute. Technical Report 941278.

Wingersky, M., Barton, M., and Lord, F. (1982). *LOGIST User's Guide*. Princeton, New Jersey: Educational Testing Service.

Using the Computer for Content Analysis

Jane C. Kronick
Susan Silver

SUMMARY. New software for the microcomputer makes formal content analysis a more accessible methodology for generating quantitative data from documents. An early program, The General Inquirer, is briefly reviewed. Four other alternatives, the use of concordances, word processing programs, software written exclusively for content analysis, and relational Data Base Management Systems (DBMS) are presented. One application of a DBMS program, DataEase, is reviewed in more detail as a program the authors have found particularly satisfactory.

Case records, field notes, unstructured interviews, and published reports are important sources of data for social work. Their use in empirically based research poses problems for social scientists generally. The researcher usually confronts an overwhelming quantity of material, the methodology is labor intensive, the decisions are difficult, and the analysis can be neither hastened nor assigned to less qualified staff. In data analysis, order is difficult to maintain, and a new

---

Jane C. Kronick holds a PhD in sociology from Yale University. On leave from the Graduate School of Social Work and Social Research, Bryn Mawr College, she is currently Director of Research at the College of Social Work, University of Tennessee, Knoxville. This article is based, in part, on experience gained while analyzing Royal Commission and Congressional hearings as part of the research funded by her multiple grants from EVIST, National Science Foundation studying cross-national policy for victims of environmental hazards.

Susan Silver holds an MSW degree from the University of Toronto. She is currently completing her dissertation at the Graduate School of Social Work and Social Research, Bryn Mawr College. The study from which she draws the examples for this article is titled "Universal Health Care: The Canadian Definition," funded by a National Welfare Fellowship from the Canadian National Department of Health and Welfare.

Requests for reprints should be sent to Jane C. Kronick, College of Social Work, University of Tennessee, Knoxville, TN 37996.

© 1992 by The Haworth Press, Inc. All rights reserved.

mountain of paper is generated. Data analysis seems to produce common feelings of boredom, uncertainty and frustration in all researchers, and most are keenly aware that many documents remain barely touched or totally ignored. New developments of microcomputer software, however, ease some of these difficulties and make document analysis a more widely acceptable research choice.

This paper (a) outlines content analysis as a basic empirical tool for document analysis, (b) contrasts it briefly with an interpretive analysis of documents, (c) reviews the early use of main frame computers for content analysis, (d) discusses some of the current microcomputer alternatives for content analysis, and (e) illustrates this method with data from a policy study.

ALTERNATIVE STRATEGIES FOR DOCUMENT ANALYSIS

Two major methodological traditions exist for document analysis: formal content analysis, and text interpretation. Content analysis is a very old technology dating back at least to the 1600's (Stone et al., 1966, pp. 22-23), but the major development occurred in the study of mass communication in the 1940's (Berelson, 1952). It is a methodology rooted in the positivistic, empirical tradition, while text interpretation reflects the hermeneutic tradition of the humanities. These two methodologies are radically opposed in underlying philosophical assumptions regarding the nature of knowledge and how it is gained.

Content analysis proceeds on the assumption that the task is to demonstrate the order hypothesized by the theory which the investigator has applied. The text, like responses to a survey questionnaire, is the index to a wider world of relationships among variables. In contrast, an interpretive approach assigns a value to the text itself in its own right. Text interpretation defines the analytic task as determining the view inherent in the text which requires preservation of text integrity. For text interpretation, the task is one of seeking understanding based on the interaction of parts with the whole while continually elaborating the context of the text (Hirsch, 1967, Gadamer, 1979). Both of these approaches can be facilitated by use of the microcomputer. We concentrate in this paper on content analysis.

CONTENT ANALYSIS AS AN EMPIRICAL TOOL

Content analysis is a technique for data transformation. It measures particular variables embedded in texts. Like all empirical research, content analysis assumes the investigator has a theory from which specific hypotheses have been generated. These hypotheses contain variables which must be measured. Content analysis differs from other empirical work primarily in the degree of difficulty in building a measurement instrument which can reliably measure the occurrence of categories on a variable within the text. Formal content analysis is a methodology for coding data within a text to measure variables.

Content analysis requires a series of decisions. Before any analysis can begin, the variables to be measured are specified by the researcher. Without this, the researcher has no direction in how to proceed. The next major decision is the definition of the unit to be analyzed. The unit can be as small as a single word or as large as a complete account of an event. In content analysis, however, once the unit is specified, it remains the unit for analysis throughout the process. As the research proceeds, the researcher is not to move back and forth between different units. The phrase is probably the most common unit for content analysis in the social sciences. Content analysis involves the building of a formal dictionary of terms which reflect the variable being measured as they occur in texts. In other words, the heart of content analysis is an elaboration of rules for coding data in texts.

Content analysis requires a sequential handling of the text. The first "pass" through the data selects sections of the text containing information relevant to the study and discards the rest. Most researchers build their "dictionaries" as the analysis proceeds. To do this, a gross categorization of information under the different variable headings is made, usually with a verbatim transcription of the material under the variable headings. This collection of information is then scanned and categories developed for each variable. The next and final step is the actual count of the occurrence of each category of each variable within the text, organized by whatever case designation the researcher has established for the analysis (client, document, interest group, etc.) As in all empirical work, the case designation is determined by the universe the researcher is studying. The final product of content analysis is carefully tabulated data which can be subjected to statistical analysis.

To summarize, content analysis is used to test hypotheses. In doing content analysis the text is destroyed, which is a legitimate activity since interest lies not in the text itself but in the text as a measure of the distribution of particular variables. The essential task of content analysis is to develop a reliable and valid method of measuring variables as they occur within a written text. Content analysis has been described as "... interaction of two processes: the specification of the content characteristics to be measured and the application of rules for identifying and recording the characteristics when they occur in the data" (Stone et al., 1966, p. 7).

For most researchers who build their own coding schemes, the process, despite the formality, requires continuous decision-making as terms used by the author of the documents are transformed into categories of specific variables. To be either reliable or valid, the directions for coding the data must be developed in detail with at least some attention paid to the context within which the terms occur. This is obvious with respect to those words which take on different meanings depending on their use, such as capital offense or capital expenditure, but many other words will have subtle differences in implication depending on the context in which they are used. The ability of the microcomputer to preserve some of the context of the words while allowing their transformation is an important asset.

THE GENERAL INQUIRER

One of the first applications of computer technology to content analysis was the development of The General Inquirer (Stone et al., 1966) at MIT. The General Inquirer is a set of programs developed for mainframe computers. In its original form, the text had to be typed onto Hollerith cards and then entered via a card reader into the computer. The programs contained initially three different dictionaries, measuring different sets of variables: The Harvard third psychosociological dictionary, The Stanford political dictionary, and the Harvard need-achievement dictionary (Stone et al., 1966, pp. 169-206.). These dictionaries are general dictionaries allowing application to a wide variety of specific research questions.

The text is entered in the computer and subjected to three separate "passes" or stages of analysis. Each is governed by a different program. In the first pass, the text is screened either by word or sentence, and information relevant to the study is tagged by comparing the material with the dictionary. The tagged data are stored in a separate file. This tagged file then becomes the data base for subsequent analysis. In the second pass, the tagged data are sorted by variable. In the third pass, the categorized data is subjected to statistical analysis. Stone et al. (1966:108-9) present a flow chart of the process.

Application of The General Inquirer to texts previously analyzed by hand demonstrates the ability of computer analysis to replicate analysis which had been carefully guided by recognized scholars. This program, however, has major obstacles to general use. Until recently the time required to type documents into the computer was itself a substantial barrier to use of the computer for this purpose. The development of text scanners like the Kurzweil scanner removes this barrier. While the text scanner is not completely reliable, the volume of text used in most computer analyses makes the occasional error of lesser importance. Also, if the microcomputer is used for text analysis, the text will be viewed repeatedly and some, if not all, of the errors of entry discovered (providing, of course, that the analyst is familiar with the documents).

In addition to the earlier difficulty of entering a text in the computer, The General Inquirer has other drawbacks. First, an adequate dictionary has to exist *before* the analysis is begun. Second, the programs are greedy, requiring both the storage capacity of a mainframe and considerable time for the continuous searching and comparing which lies at the heart of formal content analysis. Only well funded studies, therefore, make use of this software. The General Inquirer remains beyond the reach of most researchers. It has been, however, a major teaching tool regarding the process of conducting a formal content analysis since the programs identify each decision point in the analysis and its requirements. The appendix volume to The General Inquirer contains the actual programs.

OTHER OPTIONS

Four different kinds of software now exist for content analysis. All can be used on a micro-computer and thus relieve the investigator of the exorbitant costs of content analysis on a main frame.

A Concordance

One possibility is the application of a Concordance to the text. Many versions of these exist at low cost and provide the ability to extract a "key word in context" from the text upon specification of the word to be extracted. While extensive use of these has been made to build bibliographies in the social sciences (see Aldous and Hill, 1967), the major use of concordances for research purposes remains in the humanities. The advantage of these programs for research in the social sciences remains to be demonstrated (Pfaffenberger, 1988, pp. 47-50). The speed with which a concordance can move through a text and assemble all occurrences of a word in the context of surrounding phrases, however, suggests that it is a potentially very valuable asset in the analysis of the content of a text.

Word Processing Programs

Another option is to use a word processing program. For a word processing program to be useful in formal content analysis, it must allow the screen to be divided and each half scrolled independent of the other. The text being analyzed will be displayed in one half while the categories will be entered in the other half. A second requirement is the ability to "tag" the text itself by inserting markers which are references to variables identified and categorized in the bottom half of the screen. Use of this kind of program allows the researcher to read and analyze the document, line by line, selecting the material to be included in the data of the study and building the system of categories for the study as the reading proceeds. The categories of variables building on the second screen can be studied separately, and the coding process refined. The dictionary will emerge as the analysis proceeds.

The most satisfactory word processor to use for content analysis is probably Nota Bene produced for the humanities by the Modern Language Association.

This word processor has a supplementary program which permits exactly what has been described above, a split screen and a tagging capability, which allows nested and overlapping tagging so that different combinations of words within the same lines can be coded differently. The lower half of the screen allows not only the creation of categories associated with different tags, but the creation of a separate file containing good quotations or illustrative examples for the final paper. In addition, the program will count frequencies and compile a spread sheet which can be transferred to a statistical package like SPSS.

There are two major disadvantages to using Nota Bene. This is not a user friendly word processor. Like all complex word processors, it is more difficult to learn, and the basic word processor must be understood before it can be used for this purpose. Many find the documentation of Nota Bene relatively inadequate. It is fairly costly as well. For researchers familiar with this word processor, it is a highly recommended tool for content analysis. The word processing package is powerful, it has the capacity to handle languages other than English, the file construction capability supports the construction and modification of complex coding systems, and files can be formatted for automatic transfer to either SPSS/X or SPSS/PC.

The Ethnograph

Another alternative is the software packages which have been written explicitly for content analysis on the microcomputer. One such program is The Ethnograph, available directly from the authors, John Seidel and Jack Clark of the University of Colorado.

This program requires a split screen, which is split vertically with the text typed in the left side of the screen. The far left spaces are used to identify the text, with the text itself indented several spaces. As the text is typed the lines are automatically numbered. This program provides for nested and overlapping coding of the text and the creation of a code associated with each symbol used in the tagging. Similarly coded text can be extracted and printed separately allowing the researcher to review what has been done and modify the codes. For a description of The Ethnograph by the authors, see Conrad and Reinharz (ed.), 1984, pp. 110-125.

Use of the Ethnograph begins with the entry of the document into a file using only the first 40 columns. This file is converted to an ASCII file. In the next step, the Ethnograph generates a numbered file, assigning line numbers to each line. Two additional files are generated at this point, a "speaker" file and a file for "contextual comment." At this point, a copy of the numbered file is printed. Analysis begins with the printed copy. With pencil, the researcher marks off sections that are talking about specific things, the segments to be coded. These are marked in the blank right hand side of the paper. The content of these segments is then identified and labeled providing a rudimentary coding scheme. Code words are limited to ten characters. These written codes are then entered into the computer file by entering the line number to be coded and the code word, which will later appear as a symbol. At the next step, the coded file can be printed, completing the initial use of The Ethnograph. A search procedure allows all the similarly coded sections to be compiled and printed. The final part of the program allows you to interact with the text to revise and modify the coding.

The major disadvantage of The Ethnograph is its reliance on intermediary paper and pencil activities. In other words, it is not completely automated. Further, although the program uses a split screen, the tagging does not appear on the screen. You can not see what you have done, therefore, until the results are printed out. In addition, while coding the original document, you can move only forward, not backward. These characteristics of The Ethnograph are major disadvantages, making this program relatively unsatisfactory.

Despite disadvantages, the Ethnograph remains a valuable tool for content analysis. It is quite cheap to purchase, and it is easy to use. It allows the gradual development of coding schemes, allowing you to move from more general categories systematically to more specific codes by simply renaming coded material. It is a program which can provide a first taste of the reduction of tedium and the improvement in the quality of life of the researcher which occurs when the repetitive handling of text is transferred from pencil and paper to the microcomputer.

Relational Data Base Management Systems

Data base management systems (DBMS) provide researchers with a powerful tool for the storage, manipulation and retrieval of large data sets. DBMSs are structurally based using a relational, network, or hierarchical model. They are distinguished by the manner in which data are stored. In the relational model, information is stored in tables or files; in the network model the information is represented by directed graphs; and in the hierarchical model a set of trees is used to store the information. Since the early 1980s, with the introduction of microcomputers, software packages for these computers have predominantly adopted the relational model.

The popularity of relational DBMSs stems from the ease with which they can be understood and used. The user can comprehend the relational model easily since it consists of files of records and relies on familiar notions such as tables, rows and columns. The relational model closely parallels the manual use of file cards, questionnaires, tables and spreadsheets. An intuitive understanding is rapidly grasped.

The data manipulation commands (retrieval and modification demands) are uncomplicated. Only the information sought needs to be specified. Unlike queries in other models, relational commands are considered non-procedural. They do not need to include directions as to what file to access first, what index to use or which record to read first (Salzberg, 1986, p. 63).

Rapid retrieval of information in various formats and from various sources is readily accomplished by elementary commands. This facilitates aggregate operations and comparative analyses across records. Through the creation of different composite models or tables, the data can be viewed from alternative perspectives. Equally important is the relative ease with which new data can be added and existing data restructured without the need to rewrite application programs.

It is the tremendous flexibility and "user friendly" nature of the relational model that has made it an invaluable asset to both the novice and the experienced researcher.

Relational DBMSs and Content Analysis

Relational DBMSs are readily adaptable to research studies using content analysis. Given that relational DBMSs closely parallel the manual method of data collection, organization and analysis, the methodological issues inherent in content analysis must also be addressed when moving to the microcomputer. There are no new significant methodological issues introduced when adapting the study to the computer.

Content analysis requires that the integrity of the context in which the data originate be maintained. As stated by Krippendorff, ". . . any content analysis must be performed relative to and justified in terms of the context of the data" (Krippendorff, 1980, p. 23). It is the context which gives the data its specific meaning and becomes the major weapon in defending the validity of the analysis. Inevitably, a certain amount of context will be lost in the process of moving from the text to the computer/file card. Thus the main challenge for content analysis is categorizing the data in a manner that maximizes the specificity of the measures while minimizing the separation of the defining context.

Adaptation of a Relational DBMS for Content Analysis

The microcomputer, using relational database software, can be introduced at virtually any stage of research. This flexibility is due to the ease with which new information can be incorporated and existing information restructured. The sophistication with which the computer is adapted, however, is a function of the extent to which the investigator is familiar with the context from which the data will be generated. This familiarity should not be confused with the requirement that the investigator must establish a theoretical framework and a set of operationalized hypotheses to guide the analysis.

DataEase, a commercially available relational DBMS for the microcomputer, will be used as a specific example of a software program that is easily adapted for content analysis. The key features of DataEase will be illustrated using data from a study currently in progress by Susan Silver. This study, *Universal health care–The Canadian Definition*, examines the policy process surrounding the passage of the controversial Canada Health Act in 1984. The Canada Health Act prohibited physicians from "extra-billing," a practice which involved directly billing the patient above the universally established amount. Focusing on the normative assumptions that informed the positions taken by the various interest groups, the aim of this study is to arrive at a conceptual model in which the various dimensions of universal health care (equity, accessibility, responsibility, rights, efficiency) are defined and compared across the various stakeholders in the Canadian political arena.

To use DataEase for content analysis, the researcher reads the printed text and records on the microcomputer the information from the text which is relevant to the study. This material is recorded on forms in DataEase created to gather the pertinent information. The extent to which the investigator is familiar with the information will determine how precise the design of this form will be. When commencing with only a preliminary understanding of the information, DataEase can be adapted to assist the investigator in acquiring a more thorough and focused grasp of the relevant information. There is no limit on the amount of text which can be recorded in particular parts of the form.

Form #1, Canada Health Act Overview provides an example of a very basic form designed for the preliminary stage of research. This form closely parallels an open ended questionnaire. The smallest complete unit of information on the form is a field. The fields on this first form include the name of the organization, the type of organization, the key witness, etc. If the range of answers for a certain field can be predetermined, these options can be preprogrammed and displayed on the screen at the appropriate instance. For example, the "TYPE" field, which refers to the category of organization, was preprogrammed with the following five choices: medical; government; public interest group; scientist/academic; and other. This option expedites data entry and reduces the incidence of error.

When defining the characteristics or attributes of a field, DataEase is extremely flexible. A "text" field can be specified to a length of 250 characters. A "note" field allows space for multiple lines so that complete blocks of text can be entered, preserving the context.

In this example, a new record was entered for each participating organization. Next, tables of "reports" can be generated. DataEase allows one to design reports quickly and easily using the "quick report" menu. No programming is required when specifying which records to include, which fields to list, and which ways to sort and format the data. These various options simply appear as choices on the "quick report" menu.

Using the information on *Form #1, Canada Health Act Overview*, many different reports can be generated. For example, a table can be designed to display a list of organizations and their positions on the Bill. The organizations can be listed in alphabetical order, grouped by kind of organization, or grouped by position on the Bill. A "quick report" can also include a count of the number of records meeting the selection criteria. Other statistics such as the sum, the mean, the variance, and the standard deviation can be calculated for a "number"

```
FORM #1    Canada Health Act Overview
```

                                            Record Number 058

```
ORGANIZATION   :

TYPE           :Other

KEY WITNESS    :

TITLE          :

Issue Number   :00:000
```

```
POSITION ON    :  -Hospital User Fees        :
                  -Physician Extra-Billing   :
                  -Penalty:                  :
                  -Overall Position on Bill  :

MAJOR ARGUMENT:
```

```
ISSUES ADDRESSED:

1)
2)
3)
4)
5)

RECOMMENDATIONS:

1)
2)
3)
```

field. Table 1 is an example of the type of information that can be tabulated from *Form 1, Canada Health Act Overview*. Note that Table 1 is, in fact, three separate tables: one measuring position for and against extra-billing, one measuring position for and against the Canadian Health Act, and one measuring mixed positions on the two issues.

With respect to fields that include a large amount of text, DataEase allows one

Table 1: Position on Extra-Billing and on The Canada Health Act Assumed by the Interest Groups in the Opening Statements Presented at the House of Commons Hearings on the Canada Health Act

Position	Medical n=25 (%)	Government n=8	Public n=11	Academic n=6	Totals n=50
Extra-Billing:					
For-	10 (40)	3 (37.5)	0	1 (17)	14 (28)
Against-	6 (24)	2 (25)	11 (100)	5 (83)	24 (48)
Not Addressed-	9 (36)	3 (37.5)	0	0	12 (24)
Canada Health Act:					
For-	9 (36)	1 (12.5)	11 (100)	5 (83)	26 (52)
Against-	16 (64)	7 (87.5)	0	1 (17)	24 (48)
For Extra-billing AND Against the Canada Health Act	10 (40)	3 (37.5)	0	1 (17)	14 (28)
Against Extra-Billing AND For the Canada Health Act	5 (20)	1 (12.5)	11 (100)	5 (83)	22 (44)

Note: This table represents preliminary data.

to search individual records by a key word or phrase (a text string). Tables can then be generated in which fields containing the same text strings are grouped.

These preliminary reports allow the researcher to become familiar with the structure and content of the data. This new knowledge can assist with the key decisions regarding the appropriate recording units, context units, and categories for the study.

Form #2, Values is an example of a possible second stage form that builds on the information obtained from manipulating the data on the first form. Form #2 is related to Form #1 by the name of the organization. Some key or guiding issues may have been identified and the process of relating the values that inform these issues can begin. The fields called "Definition" and "Quote" allow the researcher to include a certain amount of context with which to verify the subsequent coding of values and issues into more formalized categories.

Once this second form has been completed, reports can be generated. These reports, by grouping similar values and issues, can assist the investigator in exploring various relationships across organizations, values and issues.

At this stage, formal categories can be specified. In *Universal Health Care . . . The Canadian Definition*, the investigator used the following categories of values: rights of the profession; patient rights; individual responsibility; collective responsibility; cooperative federalism; equity; and efficiency. A choice field called "Category" can be added to this second form and the value choices can be preprogrammed. For example, values such as economic freedom, professional freedom, right to reasonable compensation, indiscriminate right to practice in Medicare, etc., would be included in the category called "Rights of the Profession." These specific values demonstrate the wide, and often conflicting, operational dimensions of the more conceptual category of "Rights of the Profession."

An example of a "quick report" generated from the information recorded on Form #2, including the new field "Category," is displayed in Report I. This report groups a number of operational issues and values by the higher-level categories and lists the corresponding organizations. The next step in developing the data is the counting of items coded the same way. This produces data which can be tabulated and cross-tabulated to produce tables. Report II is an example, a cross-tabulation of two variables, values by interest group identity. The next step in the data analysis is to calculate the appropriate statistics, such as measures of association and tests of statistical significance.

In addition to these menu-driven aspects, DataEase also provides more sophisticated options. The DataEase Query Language provides the researcher with the ability to generate complex reports. Facilities are available to download data directly for use with statistical packages such as SPSS and SAS. Other features include database security and rapid backup of entered data.

In conclusion, relational DBMSs provide the investigator with a "chart" to

```
┌─────────────────────────────────────────────────────────┐
│ FORM #2: Values                                         │
└─────────────────────────────────────────────────────────┘

┌─────────────────────────────────────────────────────────┐
│  Record Number      :                                   │
│  Organization       :                                   │
└─────────────────────────────────────────────────────────┘

┌─────────────────────────────────────────────────────────┐
│  Issue          :                                       │
│  Value          :                                       │
│  Definition     :                                       │
│  Quote          :                                       │
└─────────────────────────────────────────────────────────┘
```

navigate large sets of data. With relational software packages such as DataEase, the research can progress in stages, with each stage providing a more focused view of the data. Contextual information can also be tapered as one proceeds to the more conceptual stages. As understanding increases, the task of constructing and defining "categories" for recording the data is made relatively easy. Equally important, the various stages provide the necessary evidence for defending the reliability of the coding and the validity of the conclusions.

Unlike any of the previous programs for content analysis-The General Inquirer, The Ethnograph, or word processors like Nota Bene-a data base program does not proceed from a full text first entered into the computer. While the data base program allows very flexible creation of files and subfiles and the addition of quite substantial amounts of text, the lack of access to the complete text in its original sequence on the computer can be a serious limitation, particularly when there is considerable uncertainty about what is to be coded or how the coding is to be done, or when the research requires extensive interpretation in addition to the formal content analysis.

CONCLUSIONS

This paper has presented content analysis as a method of measurement firmly located in the positivistic tradition of empirical research. It is a unique way to measure variables occurring in written texts. Content analysis proceeds according to the following steps:

REPORT I

Rights of the Profession

	Issue	Organization
1	"Reasonable and Adequate" Funding Clause Must Stay	Nova Scotia Medical Association
2	Arbitration Mechanism Sought	Manitoba Medical Association
3	Binding Arbitration Most Equitable	Manitoba Medical Association
4	CMA ... Violation of Medicare "Contract"	Saskatchewan Medical Association
5	Doctor's Indiscriminate Right To Practise In Medicare	Canadian Association of Interns and Residents
6	Doctor-Patient Rel'n As An Unwritten Contract	Quebec Medical Association
7	Doctors ... Members of Free Enterprise System	Alberta Government
8	Extra Billing ... Only Real Negotiating Tool	Nova Scotia Medical Association
9	Extra Charges and Government Control of Medicine	Prof. Eugene Vayda
10	Extra-billing : Safety Valve and Negotiating Tool	Quebec Medical Association
11	Extra-billing Guarantees Professional and Eco. Freedom	Canadian Medical Association
12	Hall 1979 Hearings ... Right To Fair Compensation	Emmett Hall
13	Med. Prof. Not A Law Unto Itself	Emmett Hall
14	Minimum Salary Guarantee From Federal Government	Quebec Federation of General Practitioners
15	Opting-Out and Protection of Economic Rights of Doctors	Canadian Anaesthetist's Society
16	Opting-Out Is A Freedom And A Symbolic Right	Ontario Government
17	Publication, "Preserving Universal Medicare" Affront To Doctors	British Columbia Medical Association
18	Right To Reasonable Compensation	Quebec Federation of General Practitioners
19	System of Merit Pay For Doctors	Ontario Medical Reform Group

Patient Rights

20	Freedom of Choice in Health Care	Canadian Association of Optometrists
21	Health Care... A Right Not A Privilege	Ontario Government
22	Health Is A Right, According To World Health Organization	Health Coalition of Nova Scotia
23	Involuntary Nature of Health	Prof. Eugene Vayda
24	Patient Rights To Access Upheld With Extra-Billing	New Brunswick Medical Association
25	Role for Voluntary Organizations	Canadian Council on Social Development
26	Stronger Consumer Role	Canadian Health Coalition

Individual Responsibility

27	Co-Insurance Fosters Responsibility and Awareness	Canadian Dental Association
28	Extra Billing ... Patient Participation Has No Adverse Effects	Alberta Medical Association
29	Extra Charges Give Consumers A Financial Stake in System	Prof. Ake Blomqvist
30	Extra Charges Promote Personal Responsibility	Alberta Government
31	Individual Responsibility Through Cost-Sharing	Quebec Medical Association
32	Market Controlled Commercial Co-insurance Required	Association of Independent Physicians of Ontario
33	Patient Participation Required	Alberta Medical Association
34	Patient Responsibility Usurped By State	Quebec Medical Association
35	Promote Cost Sharing Through Private Insurance	Quebec Medical Association

Report II: Values Introduced by Interest Groups in the Opening Statements Presented at the House of Commons Hearings on The Canada Health Act

Value	Medical N	Medical Prop.	Government N	Government Prop.	Public N	Public Prop.	Academic N	Academic Prop.
Physician's Rights	11	.24	2	.10	0	.00	2	.12
Patient's Rights	2	.04	1	.05	4	.14	1	.06
Individual Responsibility	5	.11	1	.05	0	.00	1	.06
Collective Responsibility	4	.09	2	.10	7	.24	5	.29
Equity	8	.18	3	.15	7	.24	4	.24
Efficiency	8	.18	3	.15	7	.24	4	.24
Cooperative Federalism	7	.16	8	.40	4	.14	0	.00
Total	45	1.00	20	1.00	29	1.00	17	1.01

Step 1: generation of hypotheses from formal theory
Step 2: dentification of variables for measurement
Step 3: selection of texts for analysis
Step 4: decision regarding the unit of analysis
Step 5: decisions on whether or not to sample and how
Step 6: development of simple or elementary coding scheme
Step 7: identification of parts of the text for analysis
Step 8: first pass at coding units from text
Step 9: elaboration of the coding scheme
Step 10: tabulation of results by variable
Step 11: cross-tabulation by variables
Step 12: statistical analysis of data to test hypotheses

Content analysis entails measurement of variables, identifying various manifestations of variables in a written text, and developing rules for categorizing each expression of a variable. The most simple application of content analysis will generate data in two categories: presence or absence of a variable. This is, of course, an aristotelian dichotomy to which ratio level statistics are appropriate, such as the significance of difference of proportions and other quite powerful measures.

Measurement in content analysis proceeds with the same difficulties and opportunities as measurement in any other type of empirical research. It is possible to build scales which combine information on different variables to yield either ordinal or interval data. In the example of values informing parliamentary debate in Canada, the relative incidence of values (proportion of appeals to a specific value to the total appeals to values in each submission) can be used as a ratio measure of the strength of the value for different submissions providing one is willing to accept the assumptions this decision implies.

The complexity of the value frames for different interest groups can be compiled by counting the number of different values used by each interest group, again a ratio measure. Thus, the level of measurement obtained from content analysis directly reflects the decisions made regarding how the codes are to be constructed and data used in constructing more complex measures. Just as measurement in survey research can be improved to yield higher levels of measurement so can measurement in content analysis be made more sophisticated to yield higher levels of measurement in the final data.

This paper has presented different options for automating the process of content analysis. The early major program for content analysis on the computer, The General Inquirer, was briefly reviewed. Newer options for the microcomputer have been identified with both their positive and negative features. Relational data base management systems, DataEase in particular, has been presented in more detail as a program which these authors have found particularly helpful.

The increased use of microcomputers in the execution of content analysis is important. First, the increased ease of the analysis makes content analysis a more reasonable approach to data analysis and opens more broadly the use of written records for more than illustration. The microcomputer records the decisions as they are made by the researcher, leaving a very clear trail. Inconsistency becomes obvious. Therefore, as well as facilitating analysis, it can ensure higher standards of reliability and validity to the final product. Moreover, the clarity with which content has been categorized means that studies can build on completed work, using again the same system of categorization and making only those modifications necessary to include a wider range of categories represented in additional texts.

REFERENCES

Aldous, Joan and Reuben Hill (1967). *An International Bibliography of research in Marriage and the Family, 1900-1964*. Minneapolis, Minnesota: University of Minnesota Press.

Berelson, Bernard (1952). *Content Analysis in Communications Research*. New York: Free Press.

Conrad, Peter and Shulamit Reinharz, eds. (1984). *Computers and Qualitative Data*. New York: Human Sciences Press, Inc.

DataEase International (1988). *DataEase Reference Manual*. Turnbull, CT.

Gadamer, H.G., "The Problem of Historical Consciousness" in Rabinow, Paul and William Sullivan, eds. (1979). *Interpretive Social Science a Reader*, Berkeley, CA: University of California Press.

Hirsch, E.D., Jr. (1967), *Validity in Interpretation*. New Haven, Conn.: Yale Univ. Press.

Holsti, Ole (1969). *Content Analysis for the Social Sciences and Humanities*. Reading, Mass.: Addison-Wesley.

Krippendorff, Klaus (1980). *Content Analysis, An Introduction to Its Methodology*. Beverly Hills, CA: Sage Publications.

Kronick, Jane C. (1965) *Family Life and Economic Dependency*. A Report to the Welfare Administration, Bryn Mawr, Pa.: Bryn Mawr, College.

Pfaffenberger, Bryan (1988). *Microcomputer Applications in Qualitative Research*. Beverly Hills, CA: Sage Publications.

Salzberg, Betty Joan (1986). *An Introduction to Database Design*. Orlando, Fl.: Academic Press Inc.

Seidel, John V. and Jack A. Clark (1984). *The Ethnograph*. 611 E. Nichols Drive, Littleton, CO. 80123.

Stanczyk, Stefan (1990). *Theory and Practice of Relational Databases*. London, England: Pitman Publishing.

Stone, Philip and Dexter Dunphy, Marshall Smith and Daniel Ogilvie (1966). *The General Inquirer: A Computer Approach to Content Analysis*. Cambridge, Mass.: The M.I.T. Press.

A Preliminary Examination of the Knowledge of Normative Infant Development (KNID) Inventory Using Structural Equation Modeling

John G. Orme
Judith Ann Fickling

John G. Orme earned his PhD in social work from the George Warren Brown School of Social Work, Washington University in St. Louis. Currently he is an Associate Professor of Social Work at the University of Maryland at Baltimore. His research includes applications of structural equation modeling to the measurement of parenting knowledge and to the testing of models of child abuse. Publications that complement his co-authored article in this special issue include: Hamilton, M.A. and Orme, J.G. (1990). Examining the construct validity of three measures of parenting knowledge using LISREL. *Social Service Review, 64*, 121-143; Orme, J.G. and Hamilton, M. (1987). Measuring parental knowledge of normative child development. *Social Service Review, 61*, 655-669.

Judith Ann Fickling is a PhD candidate at the University of Maryland at Baltimore, School of Social Work and Community Planning. She is also employed as a lecturer and director of the maternal and child health training project at the University of South Carolina, College of Social Work. Her current research interests are injury control and substance abuse in pregnant women. She has also conducted research in the social skills development of young adults.

Preparation of this article was supported by a Designated Research Initiative Fund grant awarded to John G. Orme from the Graduate School of the University of Maryland at Baltimore. The authors gratefully acknowledge the support provided by the School of Social Work, University of Maryland at Baltimore, the Montgomery County Department of Social Services, and Dr. Carol Peterson. Requests for reprints should be sent to John G. Orme, School of Social Work, University of Maryland at Baltimore, 525 W. Redwood St., Baltimore, MD 21201. A copy of the study questionnaire can be obtained from the senior author. The correlation matrices, the PRELIS programs used to generate these matrices, and the LISREL output (which includes the LISREL input statements), can be obtained on disk from the senior author by sending a formatted disk and a stamped return mailer.

© 1992 by The Haworth Press, Inc. All rights reserved.

SUMMARY. Structural equation modeling is a general statistical model that combines confirmatory factor analysis, multiple regression, and path analysis. It provides a comprehensive approach for testing the adequacy of measures, but virtually no applications of this approach exist in the social work literature. This article presents a new measure of parental knowledge of normative infant development, it describes the use of structural equation modeling to analyze the results of a study of 273 mothers designed to test this measure, and it discusses general considerations in the use of structural equation modeling to test measures. Results indicate that the Knowledge of Normative Infant Development (KNID) inventory measures two uncorrelated factors, early and late expectations of infant development. Each of these factors is distinct from but correlated positively with maltreating expectations, as predicted. Contrary to predictions, neither factor is correlated with family conflict.

The reliability and validity of a measure is examined by testing its performance against models derived from theory and research. Structural equation modeling is a general statistical model that combines confirmatory factor analysis, multiple regression, and path analysis, and so it is especially well-suited to testing measurement models (Byrne, 1989; Cole, 1987). This versatile approach is technically complex, but it is used widely in social science research to test measurement and causal models (e.g., Bollen, 1989; Byrne, 1989; Hayduk, 1987; Schoenberg, 1989). Almost no applications of structural equation modeling exist in the social work literature (see Hamilton & Orme, 1990 for an exception).

This article presents a new measure of parental knowledge of normative infant development, it describes the use of structural equation modeling to analyze the results of a study designed to test this measure, and it discusses general considerations in the use of structural equation modeling to test measures. The measure is named the Knowledge of Normative Infant Development (KNID) inventory, and since this is the initial report of the KNID it is necessary to briefly discuss the rationale for its development.

RATIONALE FOR THE DEVELOPMENT OF THE KNID

Evidence suggests that inadequate parental knowledge of normative infant development (birth to two years of age) may be an important determinant of ineffective parenting, and it may have adverse consequences for children and families. Inadequate parental knowledge of normative infant development has been implicated as a factor in child abuse and neglect (Azar, Robinson, Hekimian

& Twentyman, 1984), and more generally in physical punishment (Johnson, Loxterkamp & Albanese, 1982; Rickard, Graziano & Forehand, 1984), and parent/child conflict (e.g., Ticehurst & Henry, 1989). In addition, evidence suggests that parental knowledge of normative infant development is positively related to parenting skills (e.g., Stevens, 1984), positive contact with children (Chamberlin, Szumowski & Zastowny, 1979), and knowledge of child injury risks (Rivara & Howard, 1982).

Reliable and valid measures of parental knowledge of normative infant development are necessary to study the effects of such knowledge on parenting behavior and child development, to evaluate parent education programs, and to assess individual parents in a variety of settings (child welfare agencies, pediatric clinics, family counseling centers, and parent-child centers). Unfortunately, for the most part the reliability and validity of existing measures have not been examined adequately (Constable, Jacobs & Ward, 1981; de Lissovoy, 1972; Field, Widmayer, Stringer, Egnatoff, 1980; Jarrett, 1982; Kilman & Vukelich, 1985). In general, existing documentation does not support the reliability and validity of available measures (Orme & Hamilton, 1987). The one exception to this is the High Scope Knowledge of Early Infant Development (H/SED) Scale (Epstein, 1980), but in its current form this instrument primarily measures knowledge about development in the first year of life, and it was designed to be administered by an interviewer which limits its use (Orme & Hamilton, 1987; Stevens, 1984, 1989).

In addition to insufficient information about the reliability and validity of available measures of parental knowledge of normative infant development, a review of existing measures suggests that many do not include a sufficient range of content to represent this construct. Therefore, the present authors systematically constructed a new measure of parental knowledge of normative infant development, the Knowledge of Normative Infant Development (KNID) inventory, instead of further testing the reliability and validity of existing measures. The characteristics of the KNID are described below, along with the design and results of an empirical study designed to examine its reliability and validity using structural equation modeling.

METHODS

Participants

Participants were solicited for the study from mothers receiving social or medical services for themselves or their children from a county department of social services or a public health clinic in Montgomery County, Maryland, a suburb of Washington, D.C. Mothers were told that the purpose of the study was to examine their opinions and ideas about child development for normal children. A total of 273 mothers volunteered their participation, and mothers were paid $5.00 for participation.

The mean age of the mothers was 30.53 (sd = 9.50) years. The majority were black (65%), although a significant percentage was white (21%). A total of 22% of the mothers were married, 45% had never been married, and 33% were divorced, separated, or widowed. Only 19% of the mothers had less than a high-school education, 49% had a high-school education but no college, and 32% had some college education. The mothers had parented a mean of 2.35 (sd = 1.76) children (including adopted and foster children). Approximately half (51%) of the mothers had an infant living in their home.

Measures

Three scales were administered as a basis for examining the construct validity of the KNID. The Parent Opinion Questionnaire (POQ) (Azar et al., 1984) was administered to measure parental expectations of children associated with maltreatment, and the Index of Family Relations (IFR) (Hudson, Acklin & Bartosh, 1980) and the Index of Parental Attitudes (IPA) (Hudson, Wung & Borges, 1980a) were administered to measure family conflict.

The junior author and nine other interviewers administered the measures individually to the mothers. With the exception of the junior author, all of the interviewers were MSW students, and there was only one male interviewer (the female interviewers administered 80% of the measures). Most mothers completed the questionnaires themselves (90%), but the interviewers read the items to the remaining mothers.

Knowledge of Normative Infant Development Inventory (KNID)

The KNID was designed as a unidimensional measure of parental knowledge of the approximate age at which most infants acquire diverse abilities. To ensure the content validity of the measure, items were included that measured knowledge of physical, social-emotional, verbal, and cognitive abilities, although there was no expectation that these different domains measured separate identifiable constructs. To further ensure the content validity of the KNID, an extensive review was conducted of the child development literature (*Child Development, Developmental Psychology*); existing measures of parental knowledge of normative infant development (de Lissovoy, 1973; Epstein, 1980); and existing measures of general parenting knowledge (Larsen & Juhasz, 1986; MacPhee, 1981). Sources used to develop items included child psychology, pediatric, and nursing textbooks (Bornstein & Lamb, 1984; Hetherington, 1985; Wagner & Stevenson, 1982); published research on normal infant development (Capute et al., 1986; Vandell, Wilson & Buchanan, 1980); and infant care publications (e.g., Leach, 1981; Chase & Rubin, 1979). The selected items represent skills and abilities that the authors believe could be observed during typical parent/child interactions. Skills and abilities that the authors believe to be too esoteric for most parents to observe were not included (the synchronization of the infant's movements to the mother's voice).

The KNID contains 52 declarative statements (most infants can feed themselves without spilling food when they are 1 year old). Mothers are asked to respond to these statements in terms of the *average* age at which *most babies* can do different things. The mother is asked to check "agree" if she thinks that the age is about right. If she does not agree she is asked to check whether a "younger" or "older" infant could do it. If she is not sure of the age, she is asked to check "not sure" (MacPhee, 1981).

Each item is scored as correct (0) or incorrect (1), and "Not Sure" and nonresponses are scored as incorrect (the interest here is in measuring the extent of inappropriate expectations, and so inappropriate expectations were scored as 1). To minimize a response set the correct answers to the questions were distributed approximately equally among "younger" (18 items) "older" (19 items), and "agree" (15 items) responses, and items were randomly distributed throughout the questionnaire.

The correct answers for the KNID questions were determined by an exhaustive review of the empirical research concerning infant development, and each item has at least one research finding to support its correct answer. No item was included for which conflicting findings precluded a correct answer. However, cultural differences in child care practices may produce disagreement about the correctness of some answers provided by the authors.

Parent Opinion Questionnaire (POQ)

The POQ is an 80-item questionnaire with 60 scored items. It was developed to measure inappropriate parental expectations of children from infancy to 15 years, to examine differences between maltreating (i.e., abusive or neglectful) parents and other parents (Azar et al., 1984). The items for the POQ were derived from "caseworker reports of inappropriate judgments they observed in their maltreating clients which led to abuse or neglect situations" (Azar et al., 1984).

The POQ measures parental expectations in six domains, and these include "family responsibility and care of siblings," "self-care," "help and affection to parents," "leaving children alone," "punishment," and "proper behavior and feelings." Each domain is represented by 10 items. For each item, respondents indicate whether they agree or disagree with the appropriateness of the particular child behavior, and items are scored as appropriate (0) or inappropriate (1). Each subscale has a potential range of values from 0 to 10, and higher scores indicate more inappropriate expectations.

Azar and Rohrbeck (1986) reported that the 12-week test-retest reliability of the total POQ was .85, based on a sample of 16 mothers. Hamilton and Orme

(1990) reported a coefficient alpha of .87 for the total scale, based on a sample of 296 mothers. Hamilton and Orme also found, but did not report, the following coefficient alphas for the POQ subscales: family responsibility and care of siblings (.56), self-care (.58), help and affection to parents (.62), leaving children alone (.57), punishment (.60), and proper behavior and feelings (.55).

The construct validity of the POQ is suggested by Azar and Rohrbeck's and Azar et al.'s findings that abusive mothers had significantly fewer realistic expectations than nonabusive mothers. Also, Hamilton and Orme found that the POQ was correlated in the predicted manner with two more general measures of parenting knowledge and with family conflict.

Index of Family Relations (IFR)

This 25-item questionnaire was developed to measure the "degree or magnitude of problems in family members' relationships as seen by the respondent" (Hudson et al., 1980). Respondents are asked to rate each item on a five-point scale ranging from "rarely or none of the time" (1) to "most or all of the time" (5). A total score with a range from 0 to 100 is computed with higher scores indicating a more serious problem.

Coefficient alphas for the IFR have been in excess of .90 (Hamilton & Orme, 1990; Hudson et al., 1980). Strong support exists for the factorial validity of the IFR, and for its known-groups validity as demonstrated by its ability to discriminate between respondents with and without problems in family relationships (Hudson et al., 1980). Empirical support for the construct validity of the IFR has been demonstrated by its theoretically predicted correlations with a variety of variables (Hamilton & Orme, 1990; Hudson et al., 1980).

Index of Parental Attitudes (IPA)

This 25-item questionnaire was developed to measure the "degree or magnitude of a relationship problem as seen by a parent in his or her relationship with a specific child" (Hudson et al., 1980). To meet the needs of the present study, the IPA was modified slightly by changing the word "child" to the word "children" throughout the measure. The items and the total scale are scored the same as those for the IPA, and higher scores indicate a more serious problem.

Hudson et al. obtained a coefficient alpha of .97 for the IPA, and Hamilton and Orme (1990) found a coefficient alpha of .89 for the version of the IPA used in the present study. Hudson et al. provided empirical support for the factorial validity of the IPA, and for its known-groups validity as demonstrated by its ability to discriminate between parents with and without parent-child problems. Empirical support for the construct validity of the modified version of the IPA has been demonstrated by its predicted inverse correlation with parenting knowledge and its positive correlation with the IFR (Hamilton & Orme, 1990).

RESULTS

Descriptive Data

The mean, standard deviation, and coefficient alpha for the KNID, the POQ and its subscales, the IFR, and the IPA are shown in Table 1. Also, the mean percent of inappropriate expectations is shown for each knowledge measure.

As shown in Table 1, coefficient alpha is .68 for the KNID. This degree of internal consistency reliability is not acceptable for a 52-item scale. Coefficient alpha is high for the total POQ and the IFR and IPA, as found in previous research. Coefficient alpha is acceptable for the POQ subscales, given that these are 10-item subscales.

The KNID distribution is approximately normal. The IFR and IPA distributions are positively skewed with some concentration of cases at the lower end of the scale (i.e., a "basement effect"); 8% of the cases had a zero on the IFR and 3% on the IPA. The POQ and its subscales also are positively skewed, but some of these subscales had a pronounced concentration of cases at the lower end of the scale. A total of 7% of the cases had a zero on the "family responsibility" subscale, 18% on the "self-care" subscale, 20% on the "help parents" subscale,

Table 1

Descriptive Data for Scales (N = 273)

Scale	Mean	SD	Mean Percent Inappropriate	Alpha
KNID	23.89	5.79	46	.68
POQ Total	13.04	8.13	22	.88
Family Responsibility	2.46	1.72	25	.63
Self-Care	2.29	1.92	23	.63
Help Parents	2.23	1.88	22	.62
Leave Alone	1.21	1.48	12	.59
Punishment	2.10	1.92	21	.66
Proper Behavior/Feelings	2.74	1.92	27	.58
IFR	17.56	18.60	n.a.	.95
IPA	14.16	12.02	n.a.	.89

Note. n.a. indicates not applicable.

38% on the "leave alone" subscale, 24% on the "punishment" subscale, and 8% on the "proper behavior/feelings" subscale.

Exploratory Factor Analysis

The relatively low coefficient alpha for the KNID, in combination with the large number of KNID items, raises the possibility that the KNID might be measuring more than one factor. Therefore, an exploratory factor analysis was conducted to examine its factorial structure prior to examining the relationship of the KNID to other variables.

Procedure

Oftentimes the factor analysis of dichotomous items is based on the product-moment correlations among a set of items. For dichotomous items this correlation is known as "phi." However, factor loadings and the reliability of items are underestimated when phi coefficients are factor analyzed. Also, the maximum value of phi depends on item means, and this sometimes leads to the identification of factors having similar means, instead of items that measure similar domains (Muthen, 1989).

Another approach to the factor analysis of dichotomous items is to compute the intercorrelations among items using the tetrachoric correlation, and then to factor analyze this correlation matrix. However, the tetrachoric correlation is based on the assumption that the underlying variables are distributed normally. When this assumption is not met it can lead to the identification of an incorrect number of factors. Also, the tetrachoric correlation is more variable than phi, and it is difficult to compute for rare events. Nevertheless, the use of tetrachoric correlations overcomes the more serious limitations of phi because it properly recognizes the dichotomous nature of the variables (Muthen, 1989).

LISCOMP (Muthen, 1987) was used to conduct an exploratory factor analysis of the tetrachoric correlations among the 52 KNID items. LISCOMP computes weighted least squares (WLS) or unweighted least squares (ULS) estimates for dichotomous items. When it is feasible, WLS is preferable because it provides a chi-square test of model fit and standard errors of estimates, the sampling variation in the estimates is smaller, and it requires minimal assumptions about the distribution of the variables. However, ULS estimates were computed because WLS is limited to the analysis of approximately 30 variables, and it requires a minimum of 1,000 subjects when more than 10 variables are analyzed (Muthen, 1989).

An oblique rotation procedure (one that allows factors to be correlated) was used because there was no *a priori* reason to believe that the factors should be uncorrelated. The promax method was used to rotate the ULS estimates (Gorsuch, 1983).

The number of factors was determined by an examination of a scree plot

(Gorsuch, 1983, pp. 165-169; Muthen, 1989), and a consideration of the substantive interpretability of the factors. A scree plot is a graph of factors and their associated eigenvalues. A larger eigenvalue indicates that a factor is better able to account for the correlations among the observed variables. The number of factors is determined by finding the point on the scree plot at which the eigenvalues curve above a straight line formed by the smaller eigenvalues. However, the scree plot provides an estimate of the appropriate number of factors, but within the boundaries suggested by the scree plot the substantive interpretability of the factors determines the number of factors.

Results

The scree plot is shown in Figure 1. As shown in this figure, the eigenvalues curve above a straight line at the third factor. However, a much larger change in the eigenvalues occurs at the second factor. This suggests the appropriateness of a two or perhaps three factor solution.

The two and three factor solutions were computed and their interpretability examined. The proportion of inappropriate expectations for each item and the factor loadings for the two solutions are shown in Table 2.

For the two factor solution the 17 items with factor loadings ≥ .30 on the first factor each had a relatively low loading on the second factor, and each item represented *late* expectations for infant development. Item 6 is an example, and it states that "Most infants begin to walk up stairs without help when they are 2 years old." The correct answer to this item is "younger"; if a respondent answered "agree" or "older" the answer would be scored as incorrect, and it would indicate that the respondent expected this to occur later than it usually does.

The 18 items with factor loadings ≥ .30 on the second factor of the two factor solution each had a relatively low loading on the first factor, and each item represented early expectations of infant development. Item 16 is an example, and it states that "Most infants can feed themselves without spilling food when they are 1 year old." The correct answer to this item is "older"; if a respondent answered "agree" or "younger" the answer would be scored as incorrect, and it would indicate that the respondent expected this to occur earlier than it does.

As shown in Table 2, the third factor for the three factor solution has 11 items with loadings ≥ .30. All of these 11 items represented early expectations of infant development, and in general the factor loadings for these items were lower than the loadings for the items associated with the first two factors. Therefore, the third factor is represented by a smaller number of items with lower factor loadings than the first and second factors, and it seems to be an elaboration of the second factor. These results suggest that a two factor solution is appropriate.

Items with factor loadings ≥ .30 on the two factor solution were selected as indicators for each factor, and these items are marked by an asterisk in Table 2. For the first factor 17 items were selected, and for the second factor 18 items were selected. The first factor will be referred to as the "Knowledge of Normative

FIGURE 1. Scree plot of eigenvalues for tetrachoric correlations among KNID items.

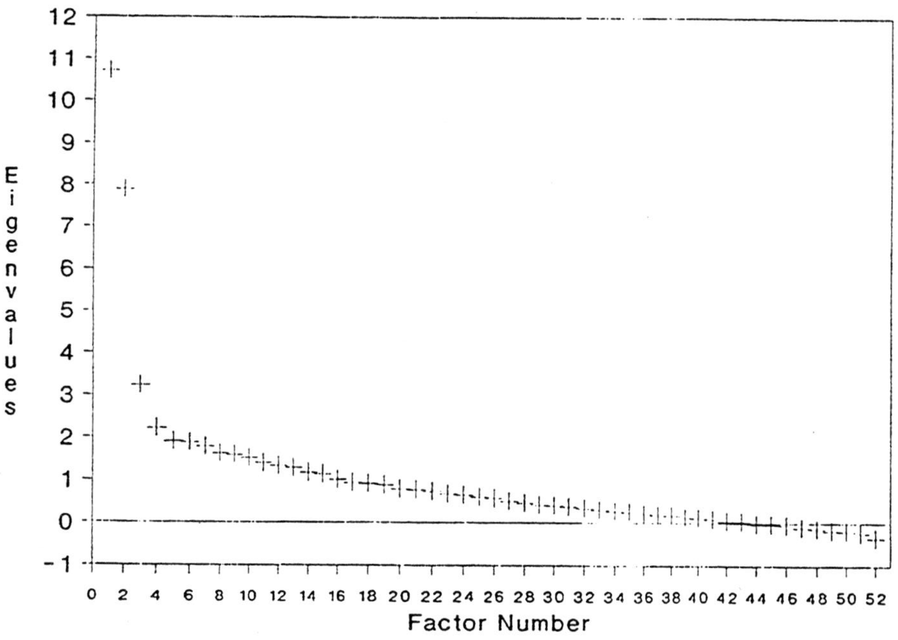

Infant Development/Late Expectations" (KNID/LE) factor, and the second factor the "Knowledge of Normative Infant Development/Early Expectations" (KNID/EE) factor.

The correlation between the KNID/EE item total and the KNID/LE item total is .00 (p = .95, two-tailed). The mean for the KNID/EE item total is 7.40 (sd = 4.24), and coefficient alpha is .83. The mean for the KNID/LE item total is 9.27 (sd = 4.46), and coefficient alpha is .86.

Table 2

Factor loadings for Unweighted Least Squares Factor Analysis of KNID Items Using Promax Rotation (N = 273)

Item	p	2-Factor Solution		3-Factor Solution		
		1	2	1	2	3
1	.26	.07	.05	.13	.06	.14
2	.23	.55*	.14	.67	.16	.24
3	.26	-.43	-.05	-.29	-.04	.38
4	.36	-.03	-.10	.11	-.09	.36
5	.51	-.03	.47*	.04	.48	.13
6	.69	.49*	-.28	.49	-.28	.00
7	.37	-.15	-.14	.04	-.12	.49
8	.77	-.19	.38*	-.20	.38	-.05
9	.33	-.67	.03	-.53	.04	.38
10	.33	-.17	-.01	.01	.01	.45
11	.96	.14	-.28	.07	-.29	-.16
12	.32	.03	.63*	.06	.63	.03
13	.38	.74*	.20	.79	.21	.08
14	.19	.15	.55*	.14	.55	-.08
15	.42	.79*	.00	.82	.01	.04
16	.25	.00	.73*	.03	.74	-.01
17	.58	.61*	-.04	.56	-.05	-.14
18	.56	.62*	-.02	.66	-.01	.08
19	.47	-.60	.10	-.52	.10	.24
20	.68	.55*	-.03	.48	-.03	-.18
21	.46	-.07	-.10	.11	-.09	.45
22	.33	-.57	.12	-.41	.13	.42
23	.21	-.02	.68*	.02	.68	.04
24	.56	-.26	.54*	-.30	.54	-.13
25	.42	.12	.62*	.06	.62	-.20
26	.55	.70*	.13	.70	.13	-.04
27	.41	.77*	.13	.86	.14	.16
28	.33	-.13	.60*	-.10	.60	.03
29	.45	-.23	-.09	-.04	-.07	.47
30	.23	.02	.74*	.06	.74	.04
31	.51	.75*	.15	.73	.15	-.08
32	.42	.61*	-.02	.64	-.02	.05
33	.40	.09	.53*	.16	.54	.13
34	.52	.14	.62*	.13	.62	-.09
35	.32	-.29	-.04	-.15	-.03	.35
36	.59	.72*	.00	.66	-.01	-.17
37	.33	-.70	.08	.59	.09	.31

Table 2 continued

		2-Factor Solution		3-Factor Solution		
Item	p	1	2	1	2	3
38	.77	.71*	-.15	.67	-.15	-.10
39	.53	.65*	-.06	.64	-.06	-.06
40	.44	.60*	.21	.69	.22	.14
41	.62	.01	.53*	-.03	.53	-.15
42	.18	.17	.68*	.23	.69	.10
43	.85	-.24	.15	-.43	.14	.44
44	.51	-.02	.62*	.00	.62	.00
45	.37	-.61	.10	-.51	.11	.26
46	.88	.45*	.03	.25	.01	-.53
47	.34	.00	.79*	-.01	.79	-.09
48	.62	.52*	.13	.52	.14	-.04
49	.50	-.05	-.22	.04	-.21	.26
50	.71	-.20	.52*	-.24	.52	-.13
51	.33	.08	.67*	.09	.68	-.04
52	.27	-.58	.09	-.41	.10	.44

Note. P indicates the proportion of inappropriate answers.

*Items selected to represent the requisite factor (i.e., items with loadings $\geq$ .30).

Confirmatory Factor Analysis

Procedure

Confirmatory factor analysis is a type of structural equation modeling that involves the construction of a hypothesized model based on theory or previous research, followed by the testing and estimation of the model (e.g., Cole, 1987; Byrne, 1989). Construction of the model first involves the specification of how factors (referred to as "latent variables") such as early or late expectations of infant development are measured by observed variables (the KNID/EE and KNID/LE items). Relationships among the latent variables, such as early or late expectations of infant development and family conflict, also are specified.

Confirmatory factor analysis is distinguished from exploratory factor analysis by the *a priori* specification of a model to be tested (Byrne, 1989; Cole, 1987). In the present study the original expectation was that the KNID would be unidimensional, and initially a model was formulated based on this assumption. However, given the results of the exploratory factor analysis the original hypothesized model was tested separately for the two KNID factors. Therefore, the procedure is not entirely confirmatory.

Figure 2 shows the hypothesized model that was tested for the KNID/EE. A separate model, comparable to the model illustrated in Figure 2, was hypothesized and tested for the KNID/LE. Separate models were tested to make sure that the ratio of the number of subjects to the number of variables was sufficient (at least a 5 to 1 ratio), and because the two factors were uncorrelated. These models were tested using LISREL (Linear Structural Relations) (Joreskog & Sorbom, 1989, PC Version 7.16), the most widely used structural equation modeling program (see Schoenberg, 1989, for a discussion of other programs).

In Figure 2 each of the boxes on the left represents an observed variable, and the ellipses represent the latent variables. One-way arrows indicate hypothesized direct influences of one variable on another. Double-headed arrows between variables indicate that these variables may be correlated, but no causal interpretation is implied. The absence of a path between two variables indicates that they are not related directly. The observed variables contain the effect of the latent variable and error variance that includes measurement error, invalid variance, and valid but unique variance; error variance is represented by the arrows to the left of each of the observed variables.

In addition to the hypothesized relationships illustrated in Figure 2, it was hypothesized that the relationship between family conflict and both early and late expectations would be stronger for parents whose children are currently infants, compared to parents whose children are older. This was hypothesized because parents with infants were contending actively with infant development, and so there would be a greater potential for inadequate knowledge to lead to family conflict. Therefore, the KNID/EE and KNID/LE models were tested separately for parents with and without infants.

To test a model such as the one illustrated in Figure 2, the hypothetical model is translated into a statistical model in which the values of certain parameters (e.g., correlations among latent variables) are estimated. Other parameters are constrained, for example by setting parameters to certain values (e.g., zero, as is implied by the absence of a path between two variables) or constraining two or more parameters to be equal.

Latent variables are not measured on any particular scale because they are hypothetical. They can be assigned any scale, but it is simplest to assign each latent variable the same scale as one of its indicators. Early expectations arbitrarily was set to have the same scale as the first KNID/EE item (item 5), late expectations was set to have the same scale as the first KNID/LE item (item 2), maltreating expectations was set to have the same scale as the family responsibility subscale, and family conflict was set to have the same scale as the IFR. The latent variables were assigned these scales by setting the raw factor loadings of these "reference" indicators to a value of one. Consequently, a unit change in a latent variable is equivalent to a unit change in the corresponding reference indicator (Hayduk, 1987). It is important to note that setting parameters equal to a value of one does not imply a perfect relationship between the observed and latent variable. Rather, a perfect relationship is indicated if the error term for an observed variable is set to zero (Herting, 1985).

As Figure 2 shows, each observed variable is constrained to load only on the

FIGURE 2. Hypothesized construct validity model for KNID/EE

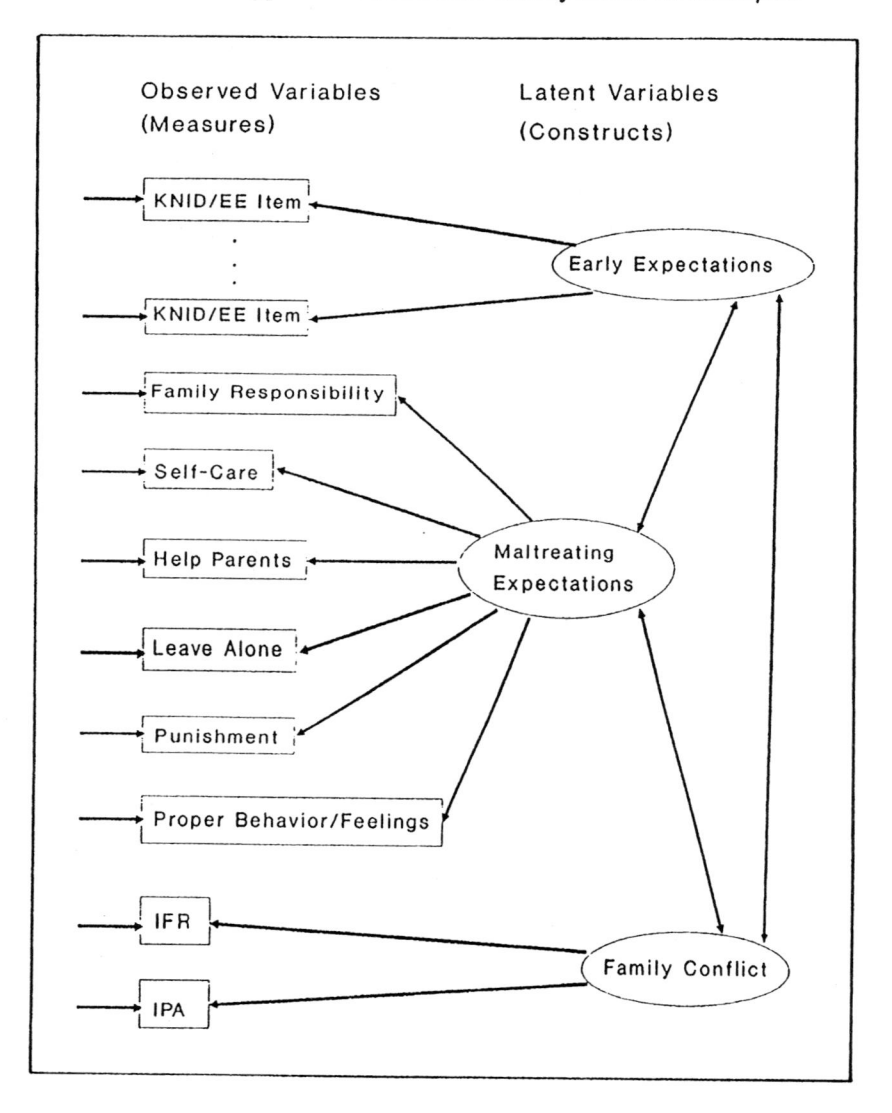

latent variable which it is hypothesized to represent; loadings on other latent variables are constrained to equal zero. Also, it was hypothesized that expectations of normative infant development (both early and late expectations) would have a positive correlation with maltreating expectations and family conflict, and that maltreating expectations would have a positive correlation with family conflict. These correlations were estimated.

Confirmation of the hypothesized relationships of the KNID/EE and KNID/LE items and latent variables would provide evidence for the construct validity of these two measures. Convergent validity of a set of observed variables (items or scale scores) hypothesized to measure the same construct is supported if the observed variables have relatively high factor loadings on the same factor (measure the same construct). Discriminant validity is supported if the observed variables have zero loadings on other putatively distinct factors (do not measure different constructs). Construct validity of observed variables is further supported if the constructs for which they are designated indicators are related in a theoretically predictable manner (Cole, 1987; Byrne, 1989).

Estimates of the "reliability" of the observed variables also are available (Bollen, 1989; Joreskog & Sorbom, 1989a). The observed variable error terms are indicated in Figure 2 by the arrows to the left of the observed variables. The complement of an error term (1-error) is an estimate of the reliability with which the observed variable measures the latent variable. These reliability estimates represent the percentage of variance in the observed variable that is explained by the latent variable. These estimates can be influenced by measurement errors, invalid variance, valid but unique variance, and by the other indicators included in a particular model. Therefore, these are lower bound estimates for the reliability of the observed variables. The error terms for the observed variables were estimated without any constraints, and the error terms were assumed to be uncorrelated.

Preparing the matrix to be analyzed. The hypothesized model implies a pattern of relationships among the observed variables. The hypothesized model is tested by comparing the implied pattern of relationships among the observed variables with the obtained relationships. The relationships among the observed variables usually are quantified by covariances or correlations, and typically the covariance or correlation matrix is computed, input, and analyzed instead of raw data (Raw data can be input directly to LISREL in some limited cases, and other types of matrices can be analyzed.)

A covariance or product-moment correlation matrix can be computed using software such as SPSS or SAS. However, PRELIS (Joreskog & Sorbom, 1988), a preprocessor of LISREL, computes a much broader array of covariances and correlations than conventional programs (e.g., tetrachoric and biserial correlations), in addition to computing standard descriptive statistics. Another advantage of PRELIS is that its output can be read directly by LISREL. Finally, PRELIS handles variables that are censored from below (a "floor effect" as indicated by a high concentration of cases at the lower end of a distribution) or above (a "ceiling effect," as indicated by a high concentration of cases at the upper end of a distribution). Therefore, given the different levels of measurement of the variables in the present study, and the fact that some of these variables were censored, PRELIS was used.

A correlation matrix was computed and analyzed instead of a covariance matrix because of the mixture of dichotomous and continuous variables. The computed matrix includes a mixture of tetrachoric correlations to quantify the relationship between dichotomous variables (e.g., the KNID items), biserial correlations to quantify the relationship between dichotomous and continuous variables (e.g., KNID items and the IFR total score), and product-moment correlations to quantify the relationship between continuous variables (e.g., POQ subscale scores and IFR total score). The tetrachoric correlation was computed for two dichotomous variables, and the biserial correlation for a dichotomous and a continuous variable because evidence suggests that these correlations provide more accurate estimates for such variables than the product-moment correlation (Joreskog & Sorbom, 1988). Finally, the POQ subscales and the IPA and IFR were specified as being censored from below in the computation of the correlation matrix.

Selecting the estimation method. LISREL provides several methods for estimating model parameters. The proposed model contains dichotomous and nonnormal continuous variables and so weighted least squares (WLS) provides the best available parameter estimates (Joreskog & Sorbom, 1989). However, WLS requires a much larger sample size than the one in the present study, and so maximum likelihood (ML) estimation was used (Bollen, 1989; Joreskog & Sorbom, 1989a). It is important to note, though, that ML assumes that the observed variables are independently sampled from a multivariate normal distribution, although there is some evidence that it is robust to the assumption of multivariate normality (Bollen, 1989; Joreskog & Sorbom, 1989a).

Testing the overall fit of a model. The hypothesized model must adequately fit the data before the parameter estimates can be interpreted (Saris & Stronkhorst, 1984). The chi-square test, the Goodness-of-Fit Index (GFI), the Adjusted Goodness-of-Fit Index (AGFI), and the Root Mean Square Residual (RMR) each provide somewhat different but valuable information about the overall fit of a hypothesized model (Wheaton, 1988). Each provides information about the degree of similarity between the observed matrix of correlations (or covariances) among the observed variables and the reproduced matrix of correlations (or covariances) generated by the hypothesized model (Bollen, 1989). If the observed and hypothesized matrices are similar, the hypothesized model cannot be rejected. However, it is important to remember that multiple models might provide equally acceptable fits (Breckler, 1990).

A large probability value for the chi-square (e.g., $p > .05$) indicates that the hypothesized model cannot be rejected. If the probability value is small (e.g., $p \leq .05$), the model does not provide an adequate fit and the hypothesized model is rejected. Therefore, in contrast to traditional significance testing, a chi-square value that is *not* statistically significant typically is preferred in testing the overall fit of a model. However, when an analysis is based on a correlation matrix rather than a covariance matrix, as in the present study, the chi-square index should be interpreted cautiously (Bollen, 1989; Joreskog & Sorbom, 1989).

Both the GFI and AGFI indicate the amount of variance and covariance explained by the total model (e.g., Cole, 1987). In general the GFI and AGFI have a potential range of values from 0 to 1, although theoretically the AGFI can be slightly smaller than 0 and slightly larger than 1 (Aneshensel, Frerichs & Huba, 1984). The difference between the GFI and the AGFI is that the AGFI adjusts for the number of parameters included in a model (e.g., factor loadings, correlations between latent variables), much like the adjusted R^2 in multiple regression (Cole, 1987). This adjustment is important because in general it is possible to obtain a better fit with more parameters. For both the GFI and AGFI, a value of 0 indicates a bad fit, and values close to 1 indicate a good fit. GFI values exceeding .90 and AGFI values exceeding .80 are generally accepted as indicating an adequate fit (e.g., Cole, 1987), although there is disagreement about standards for both indexes (Saris & Stronkhorst, 1984; Wheaton, 1988).

The root mean square residual (RMR) indicates the average absolute difference between the observed and reproduced correlations (or covariances) among the observed variables (Joreskog & Sorbom, 1989). Higher values indicate a less adequate model fit, and when a correlation matrix is analyzed it has a potential range from zero to one. Byrne (1989) suggests that when a correlation matrix is analyzed an RMR less than .05 indicates good model fit.

R^2 provides another indication of the overall adequacy of a model. R^2 indicates how well the observed variables, in combination, serve as indicators of the latent variables (Byrne, 1989; Joreskog & Sorbom, 1989).

Examining the fit of specific model parameters. The chi-square test, GFI, AGFI, RMR, and R^2 are measures for the overall fit of a model that do not indicate which part of a model is incorrect. It is possible for the overall fit of a model to be adequate, while particular relationships are specified inadequately (Bollen, 1989). Modification Indices (MI) and Standardized Residuals (SR) provide information about the adequacy with which particular parameters are specified.[1]

A Modification Index (MI) is available for each parameter that is constrained. In general, any lack of model fit results from parameter constraints, and the MI is a lower bound estimate of the expected decrease in the model chi-square value that would result if the parameter was unconstrained. Thus it indicates the improvement in fit that would result from removing the constraint on the parameter. Joreskog and Sorbom (1989a) suggest that the researcher consider releasing the constraint on a parameter with a modification index of ≥ 5 if releasing the constraint is theoretically meaningful.

A Standardized Residual (SR) is the ratio of difference between an observed correlation (or covariance) and the requisite correlation (or covariance) generated by the hypothesized model, to the asymptotic standard deviation of this difference. An absolute value greater than 2.58 indicates that the model does not adequately account for the particular correlation (or covariance) element (Joreskog & Sorbom, 1989).

Testing the comparative fit of a model. It is important to assess not only the absolute fit of a model, but its comparative fit against other plausible models (Byrne, 1989; Bollen, 1989). The statistical significance of a difference in chi-square values between different models can be used to examine the relative fit of alternative models when these models are "nested," that is if one model can be created from another model by imposing additional parameter constraints (Bollen, 1989). For example, as discussed below, a model was tested in which the correlation between maltreating expectations and early expectations was constrained to be one (this same model also was tested for late expectations). This model was compared with a model that was identical except that this correlation was estimated. A comparison of these two models provides a test of the hypothesis that the correlation between these two latent variables equals one, and as such it is a test of discriminant validity (Stacy, Widaman & Marlatt, 1990). The model in which the correlation is constrained to one is nested within (i.e., its estimated parameters are a subset of) the model in which the correlation is estimated. A nested model is more parsimonious than the model within which it is nested because it requires the estimation of fewer parameters to account for the data. Therefore, a comparison of nested models provides an indication of whether a more parsimonious model provides a comparable fit.

Nested models are compared by subtracting the chi-square value for the less restricted model from the chi-square value for the more restricted (nested) model. The difference between the chi-square values is distributed as a chi-square value. The degrees of freedom for the difference chi-square is determined by subtracting the degrees of freedom for the less restricted model from the degrees of freedom for the more restricted model (Bollen, 1989). If the probability value for the difference chi-square is sufficiently small (e.g., $p \leq .05$), the more restricted (more parsimonious) model provides a significant reduction in fit and therefore should not be accepted.

Results

Tests of model fit. Table 3 shows the tests of model fit. These results show that the early and late expectations models fit the data well for mothers with and without infants, when the correlation with maltreating expectations was unconstrained. An exception to this pattern of results is that the root mean square residual for each unconstrained model is larger than desirable (larger than .05). This may be due to the fact that ML estimation is not the ideal method of estimation for nonnormal variables. Also, for the unconstrained late expectations model for mothers without infants, the modification index was 10.30 for the constraint that KNID item 2 ("Most infants begin to turn their head in the direction of a voice when they are 9 months old") have a zero loading on

Table 3

Goodness-of-Fit Indicators for Models with the Correlation Between Knowledge of Normative Infant Development and Maltreating Expectations Unconstrained (estimated) or Constrained to 1

Models	x^2	df	p	AGFI	GFI	MI $\geq$ 5	R^2	RMR
A. Early Expectations Models								
1. Mothers With Infants								
A. Unconstrained	167.73	296	1.00	.90	.92	0	.96	.10
B. Constrained	191.26	297	1.00	.89	.90	5	.97	.24
C. 1A vs. 1B	23.53	1	.00	n.a.	n.a.	n.a.	n.a.	n.a.
2. Mothers Without Infants								
A. Unconstrained	174.86	296	1.00	.89	.90	0	.96	.11
B. Constrained	209.90	297	1.00	.87	.89	3	.97	.27
C. 2A vs. 2B	35.04	1	.00	n.a.	n.a.	n.a.	n.a.	n.a.
B. Late Expectations Models								
3. Mothers With Infants								
A. Unconstrained	134.33	272	1.00	.91	.92	0	.96	.10
B. Constrained	163.30	273	1.00	.89	.91	6	.98	.28
C. 3A vs. 3B	28.97	1	.00	n.a.	n.a.	n.a.	n.a.	n.a.
4. Mothers Without Infants								
A. Unconstrained	188.37	272	1.00	.88	.90	1	.97	.11
B. Constrained	230.27	272	.97	.86	.88	4	.98	.34
C. 4A vs. 4B	41.90	1	.00	n.a.	n.a.	n.a.	n.a.	n.a.

Note. For the above models each observed variable is constrained to load only on the latent variable that it is hypothesized to represent, no equality constraints are imposed on the loadings of the observed variables on the latent variables, and the error terms for the observed variables are assumed to be uncorrelated. AGFI = Adjusted Goodness-of-Fit Index; GFI = Goodness-of-Fit Index; MI = Modification Index; RMR = Root Mean Square Residual; n.a. = not applicable. For mothers with infants N = 139, and for mothers without infants N = 134.

maltreating expectations; this suggests that for mothers without infants this item might be an indicator of maltreating expectations. Finally, except for the unconstrained late expectations model for mothers with infants, each of the remaining unconstrained models contained one standardized residual greater than 2.58, although there was no clear pattern for these residuals.

For each model, as shown in Table 3, constraining the correlation between early or late expectations and maltreating expectations equal to one reduced the model fit. In each case the reduction in fit was indicated by a statistically significant increase in the chi-square value, an increase in the number of modification indices ≥ 5, a large increase in the root mean square residual, and a large increase in the number of standardized residuals greater than 2.58. These results indicate that there is a less than perfect correlation between early and late expectations on the one hand, and maltreating expectations on the other, and consequently that these constructs are distinct at least to some extent. This provides some support for the discriminant validity of the early and late expectations constructs. However, it also is necessary to examine the actual correlations between these constructs in order to judge fully the discriminant validity of the early and late expectations constructs and this will be done below.

Estimates of model parameters. The parameters for the hypothesized early and late expectations models were estimated for mothers with and without infants because these models provide a good fit to the data, because more parsimonious models resulted in a significant reduction in fit, and because they are theoretically meaningful. Table 4 shows the standardized loadings (correlations) of the observed variables on the latent variables and the error variance for the observed variables for early expectations. Table 5 shows the comparable information for late expectations.

The standardized factor loadings in this case are equivalent to correlations between observed variables and constructs, and as such they indicate the construct (convergent) validity of the observed variables (Aneshensel et al., 1984). (Sometimes these are referred to as "epistemic correlations.") A perfect correlation between an observed and latent variable implies that they are equivalent.

As shown in Tables 4 and 5, the correlations between KNID/EE items and early expectations, and KNID/LE items and late expectations, are moderate and acceptable, ranging from .24 to .65 (only 4 of 43 are < .30), and they are comparable for mothers with and without infants. As also shown in Tables 4 and 5, the correlations between the POQ subscales and maltreating expectations are moderate and acceptable, ranging from .37 to .56, and they are comparable for mothers with and without infants. Finally, as shown in Tables 4 and 5, the IPA is highly correlated with family conflict for early and late expectations models, and these correlations are comparable for mothers with and without infants (correlations ranging from .54 to .65). However, the correlation between the IFR and family conflict is systematically lower for mothers with infants (.39 and .37 for the early and late expectations models respectively) than for mothers without infants (.58 and .60 for the early and late expectations models respectively).

Table 6 shows the correlations among the latent variables for the early and late expectations models, as estimated for mothers with and without infants. An important characteristic of these correlations, and an important advantage of structural equation modeling, is that the correlations among latent variables are not biased by measurement error, unlike correlations among observed variables (Bollen, 1989; Joreskog & Sorbom, 1989).

Table 4

Standardized Latent Variable Loadings (Correlations) and Error Variances for Observed Variables: Early Expectations

		Mothers With Infants (N = 139)		Mothers Without Infants (N = 134)	
Variables		Latent Variable r	Error Variance	Latent Variable r	Error Variance
Latent	Observed				
I. Early Expectations					
	Item 5	.38	.86	.30	.91
	Item 8	.24	.94	.30	.91
	Item 12	.44	.80	.49	.76
	Item 14	.47	.78	.30	.91
	Item 16	.45	.80	.59	.65
	Item 23	.47	.78	.50	.75
	Item 24	.43	.81	.33	.89
	Item 25	.47	.78	.41	.83
	Item 28	.41	.83	.43	.81
	Item 30	.53	.72	.45	.79
	Item 33	.39	.85	.32	.90
	Item 34	.46	.79	.44	.81
	Item 41	.44	.81	.30	.91
	Item 42	.46	.79	.50	.74
	Item 44	.50	.75	.35	.88
	Item 47	.60	.64	.52	.73
	Item 50	.29	.91	.40	.84
	Item 51	.49	.76	.51	.74
II. Maltreating Expectations					
	Family Responsibility	.48	.78	.48	.77
	Self-Care	.54	.71	.50	.75
	Help Parents	.44	.81	.50	.75
	Leave Alone	.45	.80	.48	.77
	Punishment	.42	.82	.37	.87
	Proper Behavior/Feelings	.56	.69	.48	.77
III. Family Conflict					
	IFR	.39	.85	.58	.66
	IPA	.62	.61	.57	.68

As shown in Table 6, there is a moderate correlation between early expectations and maltreating expectations for mothers with infants (r = .61) and without infants (r = .41), as hypothesized. Similarly, as hypothesized, there is a moderate correlation between late expectations and maltreating expectations for mothers with infants (r = .44) and without infants (r = .25). The correlations between early expectations and maltreating expectations are higher (.61 and .41) than those between late expectations and maltreating expectations (.44 and .25). Also, the

Table 5

Standardized Latent Variable Loadings (Correlations) and Error Variances for Observed Variables: Late Expectations

Variables		Mothers with Infants (N = 139)		Mothers Without Infants (N = 134)	
Latent	Observed	Latent Variable r	Error Variance	Latent Variable r	Error Variance
I. Late Expectations					
	Item 2	.46	.79	.42	.82
	Item 6	.28	.92	.39	.85
	Item 13	.53	.72	.51	.74
	Item 15	.48	.77	.65	.57
	Item 17	.47	.78	.37	.87
	Item 18	.42	.82	.49	.76
	Item 20	.43	.82	.34	.88
	Item 26	.47	.78	.55	.69
	Item 27	.61	.63	.54	.70
	Item 31	.57	.68	.56	.69
	Item 32	.45	.80	.45	.80
	Item 36	.44	.80	.53	.72
	Item 38	.46	.78	.47	.78
	Item 39	.42	.82	.48	.77
	Item 40	.45	.79	.47	.78
	Item 46	.28	.92	.32	.90
	Item 48	.32	.90	.41	.83
II. Maltreating Expectations					
	Family Responsibility	.46	.78	.48	.77
	Self-Care	.49	.76	.45	.80
	Help Parents	.46	.79	.53	.72
	Leave Alone	.51	.74	.49	.76
	Punishment	.44	.80	.38	.86
	Proper Behavior/Feelings	.53	.72	.49	.76
III. Family Conflict					
	IFR	.37	.86	.60	.63
	IPA	.65	.57	.54	.71

correlations between early expectations and late expectations on the one hand, and maltreating expectations on the other, are higher for mothers with infants (.61 and .44) than for mothers without infants (.41 and .25). Finally, the correlation of .61 between early and maltreating expectations for mothers without infants suggests substantial overlap in these constructs for this population.

Contrary to predictions, early expectations is not correlated with family conflict for mothers with infants (r = .16) or without infants (r = .06), and late

Table 6

Correlations Among Latent Variables

A. Early Expectations

Latent Variables	Early Expectations	Maltreating Expectations	Family Conflict
Early Expectations	1.00	.61	.16
Maltreating Expectations	.41	1.00	.41
Family Conflict	.06	.23	1.00

B. Late Expectations

Latent Variables	Late Expectations	Maltreating Expectations	Family Conflict
Late Expectations	1.00	.44	.17
Maltreating Expectations	.25	1.00	.41
Family Conflict	-.06	.22	1.00

Note. Correlations above the main diagonal are for mothers with infants (N = 139), and correlations below the main diagonal are for mothers without infants (N = 134).

expectations is not correlated with family conflict for mothers with infants (r = .17) or without infants (r = -.06). Also, maltreating expectations is not correlated with family conflict except for the early expectations model for mothers without infants (r = .41).

DISCUSSION

The results of an exploratory factor analysis of the KNID suggest that it measures two uncorrelated factors, early and late expectations of infant development. Two non-overlapping subsets of items were identified as indicators for each of these factors, and the construct validity of each of these two subsets was tested. Results for the early expectations factor provided support for a model in which the early expectations items loaded on early expectations but not on maltreating expectations or family conflict, and early expectations was distinct from but positively correlated with maltreating expectations. Comparable results were obtained for the late expectations factor. Results did not support the hypotheses that early and late expectations are correlated positively with family conflict for mothers with infants.

These results should be tempered by a consideration of the characteristics of the sample on which they are based. The sample included mothers but not fathers. Most of the mothers were single parents (77%) who were receiving social or medical services from a department of social services or a public health clinic. Most mothers (81%) had at least a high school education. The validity of the KNID/EE and KNID/LE might be different when administered to fathers, less educated parents, or maltreating parents, and future research should examine the validity of the KNID/EE and KNID/LE with different relevant samples.

Results in the present study should be viewed tentatively for two additional reasons. First, the early and late expectations factors were unexpected and were discovered using exploratory factor analysis. Therefore, it is important to replicate the presence of these seemingly distinct factors using strictly confirmatory procedures. Second, in order to ensure a sufficient subject to variable ratio the validity of these two factors was estimated separately. It is possible that the parameter estimates would be different if the validity of both factors was estimated jointly, and future studies should include sufficient sample sizes to test such a model.

Greater diversity in the type of validity information available for the KNID/EE and KNID/LE also is necessary if these measures are to be used with confidence. For example, evidence of the known-groups validity of these measures would be useful (e.g., differences between child development specialists and mothers from the general population). The theoretical network in which these measures are embedded also should be expanded, and these theoretical relationships empirically tested. This network might include, for example, variables hypothesized to lead to the development of early and late expectations of infant development (e.g., previous experiences with different types of children, parental aspirations for their children, completion of parenting education classes), and variables hypothesized to result from early and late expectations of infant development (rate of child development, parental stress, discipline problems, home injuries to children).

Structural equation modeling provides a comprehensive statistical framework for such empirical tests of measurement models, as illustrated in the present study. Moreover, structural equation modeling is not limited to tests of measurement models (Bollen, 1989; Lavee, 1988; Joreskog & Sorbom, 1989). It merges confirmatory factor analysis, path analysis, and regression analysis, and so it has a variety of general uses. For example, structural equation modeling is used most widely to test causal path analysis models at the level of latent variables. One major advantage of this is that with latent variable path models, measurement error does not bias the estimates of causal influences, unlike traditional path analysis and regression analysis with observed variables. Structural equation modeling also is useful for estimating longitudinal models because it can accommodate correlated errors, and it can be used to estimate between group mean differences at the level of latent variables (ANOVA and ANCOVA models).

Structural equation modeling does have limitations. For example, it is possible to test models with different types of nonnormal variables using programs such as LISCOMP, or LISREL used in conjunction with PRELIS. However, the preferred estimator for testing models with nonnormal variables (i.e., WLS) is limited to models with fewer variables and much larger sample sizes than estimators for normal variables (Joreskog & Sorbom, 1989; Muthen, 1989; Tanaka, 1987). Another limitation of structural equation modeling is that in general it is difficult to estimate complex linear and interactive effects, although this is possible. Finally, in addition to the statistical complexities involved in testing and interpreting structural equation models, the computer software required to estimate these models is unfamiliar to most social work researchers and it is not simple to master. However, recent software has simplified the programming tasks (Bentler, 1989; Joreskog & Sorbom, 1987; Steiger, 1989), and the documentation for programs such as LISREL, EQS, and LISCOMP provides a wealth of examples.

The advantages of structural equation modeling for testing measurement and causal models far outweigh the limitations. Consequently, structural equation modeling deserves much wider use by social work researchers.

NOTE

1. In addition to examining the extent to which particular relationships are specified adequately LISREL provides "t-values" for each estimated parameter that can be used to test the hypothesis that a population parameter is zero. However, when an analysis is based on a correlation matrix instead of a covariance matrix, as in the present study, the t-values are incorrect and should not be used.

REFERENCES

Aneshensel, C. S., Frerichs, R. R., & Huba, G. J. (1984). Depression and physical illness: A multiwave, nonrecursive causal model. *Journal of Health and Social Behavior, 25*, 350-371.

Azar, S. T., Robinson, D. R., Hekimian, E., & Twentyman, C. T. (1984). Unrealistic expectations and problem-solving ability in maltreating and comparison mothers. *Journal of Consulting and Clinical Psychology, 52*, 687-691.

Azar, S. T., & Rohrbeck, C. A. (1986). Child abuse and unrealistic expectations: Further validation of the Parent Opinion Questionnaire. *Journal of Consulting and Clinical Psychology, 54*, 867-868.

Bentler, P. M. (1985). *Theory and implementation of EQS, a structural equations program.* Los Angeles: BMDP Statistical Software.

Bentler, P. M. (1989). *EQS structural equations program manual.* Los Angeles: BMDP Statistical Software.

Bentler, P. M. (1990). Comparative fit indexes in structural models. *Psychological Bulletin, 107*, 238-246.

Bollen, K. A. (1989). *Structural equations with latent variables.* New York: John Wiley & Sons.

Bornstein, M. H., & Lamb, M. E. (1984). *Developmental psychology: An advanced textbook.* Hillsdale, NJ: Lawrence Erlbaum.

Breckler, S. J. (1990). Applications of covariance structure modeling in psychology: Cause for concern? *Psychological Bulletin, 107*, 260-273.

Byrne, B. M. (1989). *A primer of LISREL: Basic applications and programming for confirmatory factor analytic models.* New York: Springer-Verlag.

Capute, A. J., Palmer, F. B., Shapiro, B. K., Wachtel, R. C., Schmidt, S., & Ross, A. (1986). Clinical Linguistic and Auditory Milestone Scale: Prediction of cognition in infancy. *Developmental Medicine and Child Neurology, 28*, 762-771.

Chamberlin, R. W., Szumowski, E. K., Zastowny, T. R. (1979). An evaluation of efforts to educate mothers about child development in pediatric office practices. *American Journal of Public Health, 69*, 875-886.

Chase, R. A., & Rubin, R. R. (Eds.) (1979). *The first wondrous year.* New York: Macmillan.

Cole, D. A. (1987). Utility of confirmatory factor analysis in test validation research. *Journal of Consulting and Clinical Psychology, 55*, 584-594.

Constable, E., Jacobs, E., & Ward, A. (1981). Test for measuring parents' knowledge and expectations of early childhood development. *Perceptual and Motor Skills, 52*, 82.

de Lissovoy, V. (1973). High school marriages: A longitudinal study. *Journal of Marriage and the Family, 35*, 245-255.

Epstein, A. S. (1980). *Assessing the child development information needed by adolescent parents with very young children.* Ypsilanti, MI: High/Scope Educational Research Foundation.

Field, T. M., Widmayer, S. M., Stringer, S., & Ignatoff, E. (1980). Teenage, lower-class, black mothers and their preterm infants: An intervention and developmental follow-up. *Child Development, 51*, 426-436.

Gorsuch, R. L. (1983). *Factor analysis* (2nd ed.). Hillsdale, NJ: Lawrence Erlbaum.

Hamilton, M. A., & Orme, J. G. (1990). Examining the construct validity of three measures of parenting knowledge using LISREL. *Social Service Review, 64*, 121-143.

Hayduk, L. A. (1987). *Structural equation modeling with LISREL: Essentials and advances.* Baltimore: The Johns Hopkins University Press.

Hetherington, E. M. (Ed.) (1985). *Review of child development research* (Vol. 5). Chicago: University of Chicago Press.

Hudson, W. W., Acklin, J. D., & Bartosh, J. C. (1980). Assessing discord in family relationships. *Social Work Research and Abstracts, 21*-29.

Hudson, W. W., Wung, B., & Borges, M. (1980a). Parent-child relationship disorders: The parent's point of view. *Journal of Social Service Research,* 283-294.

Johnson, C. F., Loxterkamp, D., & Albanese, M. (1982). Effect of high school students' knowledge of child development and child health on approaches to child discipline. *Pediatrics, 69,* 558-563.

Joreskog, K. G., & Sorbom, D. (1987). *SIMPLIS: A simplified version of LISREL.* Mooresville, IN: Scientific Software, Inc.

Joreskog, K. G., & Sorbom, D. (1988). *PRELIS: A program for multivariate data screening and data summarization* (2nd ed.). Mooresville, IN: Scientific Software, Inc.

Joreskog, K. G., & Sorbom, D. (1989). *LISREL 7: A guide to the program and applications* (2nd ed.). Chicago: SPSS.

Joreskog, K. G., & Sorbom, D. (1989a). *LISREL 7: User's reference guide.* Mooresville, IN: Scientific Software, Inc.

Kilman, D. S., & Vukelich, C. (1985). Mothers and fathers: Expectations for infants. *Family Relations, 34,* 305-313.

Larsen, J. J., & Juhasz, A. M. (1986). The Knowledge of Child Development Inventory. *Adolescence, 21,* 39-54.

Lavee, Y. (1988). Linear structural relationships (LISREL) in family research. *Journal of Marriage and the Family, 50,* 937-948.

Leach, P. (1981). *Your baby and child: From birth to age five.* New York: Alfred A. Knopf.

MacPhee, D. (1981). *Knowledge of Infant Development manual.* Unpublished manuscript, University of North Carolina, Department of Psychology, Chapel Hill.

Muthen, B. (1987). *LISCOMP Analysis of linear structural equations with a comprehensive measurement model.* User's Guide. Mooresville, IN: Scientific Software.

Muthen, B. (1989). Dichotomous factor analysis of symptom data. In W. Eaton and G. Bohrnstedt (Eds.), Latent variable models for dichotomous outcomes: Analysis of data from the Epidemiological Catchment Area Program. *Sociological Methods and Research, 18,* 19-65.

Orme, J. G., & Hamilton, M. (1987). Measuring parental knowledge of normative child development. *Social Service Review, 61,* 655-669.

Rickard, K. M., Graziano, W., & Forehand, R. (1984). Parental expectations and childhood deviance in clinic-referred and non-clinic children. *Journal of Clinical Child Psychology, 13,* 179-186.

Rivara, F. P., & Howard, D. (1982). Parental knowledge of child development and injury risks. *Developmental and Behavioral Pediatrics, 3*, 103-105.

Saris, W. E., & Stronkhorst, L. H. (1984). *Causal modelling in nonexperimental research*. Amsterdam: Sociometric Research Foundation.

Schoenberg, R. (1989). Covariance structure models. *Annual Review of Sociology, 15*, 425-440.

Stacy, A. W., Widaman, K. F., Marlatt, G. A. (1990). Expectancy models of alcohol use. *Journal of Personality and Social Psychology, 58*, 918-928.

Steiger, J. H. (1989). *EzPath causal modeling: A supplementary module for SYSTAT and SYGRAPH*. Evanston, IL: SYSTAT.

Stevens, J. H., Jr. (1984). Child development knowledge and parenting skills. *Family Relations, 33*, 237-244.

Stevens, J. H., Jr. (1989). Shared Knowledge about infants among fathers and mothers. *Journal of Genetic Psychology, 149*, 515-525.

Tanaka, J. S. (1987). "How big is big enough?": Sample size and goodness of fit in structural equation models with latent variables. *Child Development, 58*, 134-146.

Ticehurst, R. L., & Henry, R. L. (1989). Stage-related behavioural problems in the 1-4 year old child: Parental expectations in a child development unit referral group compared with a control group. *Australian Paediatric Journal, 25*, 39-42.

Vandell, D. L., Wilson, K. S., & Buchanan, N. R. (1980). Peer interaction in the first year of life: An examination of its structure, content, and sensitivity to toys. *Child Development, 51*, 481-488.

Wagner, D. A., & Stevenson, H. W. (Eds.) (1982). *Cultural perspectives on child development*. San Francisco: W. H. Freeman.

Wheaton, B. (1988). Assessment of fit in overidentified models with latent variables. In J. S. Long (Ed.), *Common Problems/Proper Solutions: Avoiding Error in Quantitative Research* (pp. 193-225). Beverly Hills, CA: Sage.

The Use of Logistic Regression in Social Work Research

Nancy Morrow-Howell
Enola K. Proctor

SUMMARY. Many dependent variables of interest to social work researchers are dichotomous rather than continuous, and an appropriate and powerful statistical procedure for modeling such variables is logistic

---

Nancy Morrow-Howell is Assistant Professor and Coordinator of the Gerontology concentration at the George Warren Brown School of Social Work, Washington University in St. Louis. Dr. Morrow-Howell completed her doctoral work at the University of California, Berkeley, CA. Her research interests are in home care for the elderly. She has published two related papers: Proctor, E. and Morrow-Howell, N. (1990). Complications in discharge planning. *Health and Social Work*, 15 (1), 45-54; Morrow-Howell, N., Proctor, E. and Mui, A. (1991). Adequacy of discharge plans for elderly patients. *Social Work Research and Abstracts*, 27 (1), 6-13.

Enola K. Proctor is Professor and Chair, PhD Program in Social Work at the George Warren Brown School of Social Work, Washington University. She earned her PhD from Washington University. Her current research addresses outcomes of health and mental health practice, as well as the impact of race, gender and socioeconomic factors. She has published two related papers: Proctor, E. and Morrow-Howell, N. (1990). Complications in discharge planning. *Health and Social Work*, 15 (1), 45-54; Morrow-Howell, N., Proctor, E. and Mui, A. (1991). Adequacy of discharge plans for elderly patients. *Social Work Research and Abstracts*, 27 (1), 6-13.

This paper was presented at the 1990 Annual Program Meeting of the Council on Social Work Education in Reno, NV in March, 1990 at a Symposium titled "Quantitative Methods in Social Work Research." Data reported in this paper were collected in a study funded by grant number HS05804 from the Agency for Health Care Policy and Research, Public Health Service; by an award from the AARP Andrus Foundation; and by a Faculty Research Award from The George Warren Brown School of Social Work. Requests for reprints should be sent to Nancy Morrow-Howell, George Warren Brown School of Social Work, Washington University, St. Louis, MO 63130.

© 1992 by The Haworth Press, Inc. All rights reserved.

regression. This paper presents the assumptions of logistic regression; the estimation procedure; the testing and interpretation of parameters; and measures of the goodness of the model. A review of recent social work research which utilizes the procedure is included.

Many dependent variables of interest to social work researchers are dichotomous rather than continuous. Examples include recidivism, the occurrence of a particular diagnosis, use of service, hospital readmission, compliance, suicide, and family dissolution. A powerful statistical procedure for modeling such dependent variables is logistic regression, a variant of traditional multiple regression suited for binary response variables and continuous independent variables. Although the procedure was introduced almost thirty years ago, only recently have computer software packages made it widely available (Cox, 1977). Logistic regression is frequently used by economists and epidemiologists, but it is infrequently used by social work researchers. Since it is often the most appropriate approach with dichotomous variables, the technique should be familiar to social work researchers so that their work keeps pace with improvements in the field of statistical analyses.

This paper is aimed at increasing knowledge about logistic regression among social work researchers. Six topics will be presented: (1) the assumptions of logistic regression; (2) the dependent variable to be estimated; (3) the maximum likelihood estimation procedure; (4) testing and interpreting the significance of parameter estimates; (5) the goodness of the model; and (6) appropriate choice of the procedure. Finally, use of logistic regression in the current social work literature is evaluated.

Salient points will be demonstrated with examples from the authors' research on hospital discharge planning for Medicare patients. Readmission information was collected one month post-discharge for 361 patients. If a patient returned to the hospital at any time during the first month post-discharge, readmission was coded as 1; if the patient remained in the community during that time period, readmission was coded as 0. There were 71 readmissions and 290 non-readmissions. Because the dependent variable is binary and particularly because the incidence of readmission is only 20%, logistic regression is the appropriate procedure to identify patient characteristics associated with readmission.

Three patient variables are tested in a logistic regression model: diagnosis of congestive heart failure (CHF) versus other diagnoses in the study (i.e., hip fracture and cerebral vascular accidents); gender; and functional dependency. A patient was coded as 1 if the primary diagnosis was CHF. Females were coded as 1. Functional dependency ranged from 0 to 24 with higher scores representing a more debilitated physical condition at discharge. As with ordinary least squares (OLS) regression, both dummy and continuous variables can be used in logistic regression. In fact, as Morgan and Teachman (1988) point out, the term logistic regression is used when one or more of the independent variables are continuous, and the term logit reserved for cases where all predictor variables are nominal level. Table 1 presents the computer output of the SAS logistic regression procedure. This output will be referred to throughout the paper to illustrate various points. Sample size, distribution of the dependent variable, and descriptive statistics on the independent variables are displayed at the top of the output.

THE ASSUMPTIONS OF LOGISTIC REGRESSION

Logistic regression is a type of log-linear analysis used with a binary dependent variable (Knoke and Burke, 1980). Logistic regression can also be

TABLE 1

SAS

LOGISTIC REGRESSION PROCEDURE

DEPENDENT VARIABLE: READMIT

361	OBSERVATIONS
290	READMIT = 0
71	READMIT = 1
35	OBSERVATIONS DELETED DUE TO MISSING VALUES

VARIABLE	MEAN	MINIMUM	MAXIMUM	S.D.
CHF	0.260388	0	1	0.439455
DEPENDENCY	13.5623	0	24	5.99047
GENDER	0.759003	0	1	0.428282

-2 LOG LIKELIHOOD FOR MODEL CONTAINING INTERCEPT ONLY=357.94

MODEL CHI-SQUARE=10.97 3 D.F. (SCORE STAT.)   P=0.0119.
CONVERGENCE IN 5 ITERATIONS WITH 0 STEP HALVINGS R=0.119.
MAX ABSOLUTE DERIVATIVE=0.2131D-09.   -2 LOG L=346.88.
MODEL CHI-SQUARE=11.06 WITH 3 D.F. (-2 LOG L.R.) P=0.0114.

VARIABLE	BETA	STD. ERROR	CHI-SQUARE	P	R
INTERCEPT	-2.75929640	0.49820691	30.67	0.0000	
CHF	0.76289153	0.29958276	6.48	0.0109	0.112
DEPENDENCY	0.05587833	0.02334368	5.73	0.0167	0.102
GENDER	0.44262969	0.33598738	1.74	0.1877	0.000

C=0.622   SOMER DYX=0.243   GAMMA=0.254   TAU-A=0.07

used with dependent variables with more than two categories, but binary variables are the focus of this paper. Logistic modeling is based on the assumption that the underlying relationship between the dependent and independent variables is a slanted S-shaped function called a sigmoid curve. The values for the dependent variable are presented as probabilities that range between 0 and 1 with the maximum slope of the curve in the mid-range (see Figure 1). This implies that the independent variable has its greatest impact at some midpoint, where the slope of the curve is the greatest, and less impact at the ends of the range where the slope of the sigmoid curve is smaller. This assumption differs from that of OLS regression where the relationship is considered linear and the impact of an independent variable is seen as constant over the total range of values.

In logistic regression, a model is fit to the binary dependent variable based on the assumption:

$$\text{Prob } (Y = 1) = 1/[1 + e^{-(B_0 + B_1X_1 + \ldots B_pX_p)}] \qquad \text{Formula (1)}$$

That is, the probability of any particular observation being in the category coded as 1 can be calculated by using the coefficients in the model (the B's), the actual values of the independent variables (the X's) on that observation, and the value of the constant e-a non-terminating, non-repeating decimal which to five significant figures is 2.7182. The model is termed log-linear because the constant e is the base of the natural logarithm and is raised to a power which is a linear function. As shown in the equation above, $-(B_0 + B_1X_1 + \ldots B_pX_p)$ is a natural logarithm expressed as a linear function.

As seen in Formula 1, as the value of an independent variable changes, the value of the exponent changes, and the change in the dependent variable (that is, the change in probability) is exponential. Thus the logistic function is nonlinear, and a unit change in an independent variable has a different impact on the dependent variable at different values of the independent variable. Consequently, the effect of an independent variable must be evaluated at several points to understand its relationship to the dependent variable (Cleary and Angel, 1984).

THE DEPENDENT VARIABLE TO BE ESTIMATED

In an analysis where the dependent variable is binary, the observed dependent variable assumes one of two values, 0 and 1 in the readmission example. These observed values are used in a model fitting process that yields predicted values which are continuous numbers between 1 and 0. These predicted values are interpreted as the probability of being in category 1. In the example, the dependent variable is thus the probability of being readmitted.

This probability can also be stated in terms of odds: the odds of being in the first category (readmitted) rather than the second (not readmitted). From prob-

Figure 1: The Logistic Function: Sigmoid or S-Shaped Model

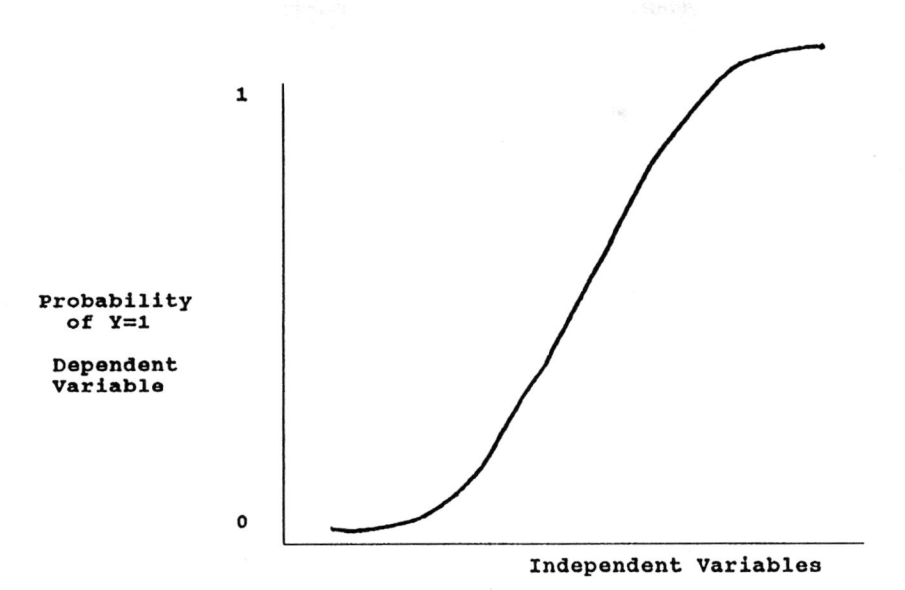

[Graph: Probability of Y=1 (Dependent Variable) on vertical axis from 0 to 1, Independent Variables on horizontal axis, showing an S-shaped curve]

ability, odds can be easily calculated: odds = P/(1-P). Thus, in the readmission example, if an individual has a .35 probability of being readmitted, the odds of being readmitted are .35/(1-.35) or .54.

Exactly the same information as in the probability and the odds is contained in the natural logarithm of the odds or the log odds. This term is called the logit of P, that is, the log of the odds of falling into one group as opposed to the other. The odds of .54 of readmission (the same as a .35 probability of being readmitted) can be expressed as a natural log. The natural log of .54, is -.62. Thus e raised to the power of -.62 equals .54 ($e^{-.62} = .54$). The dependent variable expressed in terms of log odds (-.62) can be represented by a linear model (ln odds = $a+b_1X_1+b_2X_2+b_3X_3$) (Cox, 1977; Everitt, 1977).

Thus, parameter estimates on the independent variables are calculated (as discussed below) and used to produce expected values of the log odds. Odds and probabilities can both be calculated from the log odds. (See Note 2 for calculation of the dependent variable readmission in terms of log odds, odds, and probability.) Because the log odds is an exponent, both odds and probability change in a non-linear fashion as the values of the independent variables vary. When calculated as probabilities, the predicted values vary between 0 and 1.

ESTIMATING THE MODEL
WHICH FITS THE DEPENDENT VARIABLE

In logistic regression, maximum likelihood estimation (MLE) procedures use the observed values of 1 and 0 on the dependent variable to estimate coefficients for the independent variables in the model. The principle of MLE is to choose coefficients which maximize the likelihood of observing the particular Y value. Several coefficient values are tried until the likelihood value is maximized. Conceptually, OLS and MLE differ. While OLS chooses coefficients associated with the smallest sum of squared errors in the fit between the model and data, MLE chooses coefficients associated with the highest probability or likelihood of obtaining the observed Y values (Aldrich and Nelson, 1984). Also, while OLS procedures involve the algebraic solution to a set number of equations (the normal equations), there is not a single set of equations derived from MLE estimation; instead approximations by standard iterative algorithms are used. Estimates are changed incrementally until convergence is obtained. This computer process is time-consuming and expensive. When convergence is never obtained or requires an extremely large number of iterations, there are probably too few numbers in the sample size or too many independent variables to be estimated (Walsh, 1987).

As shown in Table 1, SAS reports the number of iterations required for convergence of the estimates; in estimating the parameters for the readmission example, 5 iterations were needed. At the bottom of Table 1, the coefficients (betas) and the standard errors resulting from the estimation procedures are presented.

TESTING THE SIGNIFICANCE OF THE PARAMETERS

Two ways are generally used to test the statistical significance of the estimated parameters: (1) the MLE chi-square statistic (Wald statistic) and (2) the coefficient to standard error ratio (coeff/s.e.). Both tests are comparable, as the Wald statistic is calculated by dividing the coefficient estimate by its standard error and squaring the result (Harrel, 1983). In Table 1, the SAS output presents the Wald statistic for each independent variable in the column labeled chi-square. Probability levels associated with the test statistic are given. The ratio of the parameter estimate over its standard error (not given in SAS output) can be evaluated using the t-distribution, and a probability level can be ascertained (Engelman, 1983). When the ratio approaches 2, there is a case for statistical significance.

Another approach to testing the significance of an independent variable is to run two models, one which includes the variable and one which does not. The difference between the chi-squares for the two models represents the change due to the effect of the individual variable being tested. This difference follows the chi-square distribution under the assumption that the actual value equals 0, the null hypothesis (df = 1).

In the readmission example, chi square values indicate that the effects of two independent variables reach statistical significance: diagnosis of CHF and functional dependency. The effect of gender is not significant.

INTERPRETING THE ESTIMATED PARAMETERS

One level of interpretation is calculating the probability that any particular observation is in category one. Using Formula 1 from above, one can calculate the probability of readmission for a female patient with the diagnosis of congestive heart failure and a dependency score of 8. The probability of readmission for such a patient is .25 (see Note 1). The calculation of probabilities should use critical values of the independent variables that have particular significance. For example, calculations at the mean of an independent variable and at one standard deviation above and below the mean give substantively important information about the impact of an independent variable as its values change (Cleary and Angel, 1984). Results usually take the form of a table which presents various values of the independent variables and the associated probabilities.

Another level of interpretation involves estimating the effects of the various independent variables. The direction of the relationship as well as the magnitude of the relationship are of interest, as in OLS regression. In logistic regression, the direction of the relationship is indicated by the sign on the parameter estimate. Thus, the positive sign on the estimate of the functional dependency measure means that as the dependency of the patient increases, the probability of readmission increases.

Understanding the magnitude of the relationship is less straightforward. Indeed, the appeal of OLS regression is the direct interpretation of a coefficient as the amount of change in the dependent variable associated with a unit change in the independent variable, holding the values of the other independent variables constant. Similar interpretations of the coefficients calculated in logistic regression are also possible. Since b_1 represents a change in the log odds associated with a unit change in X_1, an additive change in the log odds represents a exponential or multiplicative change in the odds or probability of the dependent variable being in one category.

Using the changes in the log odds associated with an independent variable, interpretations about the effects of that variable can be made. From Formula 1, it can be shown that the quantity e^{b_1} is the estimated odds ratio associated with a unit change in X_1, controlling for all other variables in the model (Fleiss, 1981). The exponent b_1 can be multiplied by any change of interest in the independent variable to determine the change in the odds (i.e., the odds ratio) associated with that change. For example, b_1 could be multiplied by 10 to see the effect of a 10 point change in the independent variable, functional dependency, on the odds of readmission. This effect is called the odds ratio since it is a ratio of two odds-the odds of readmission for two patients identical except that one patient's functional dependency score is ten points higher.

The odds ratios are not part of the SAS output and must be calculated, but this calculation is quite simple. In the discussion that follows, examples of interpreting odds ratio will be shown for two dichotomous independent variables-one statistically significant and one not-and for a continuous independent variable.

In the readmission example, one can interpret the effect of CHF diagnosis, a dichotomous variables that is significantly related to readmission. By calculating e^b or in this case, $e^{.76}$, a value of 2.13 is obtained. Thus, the odds of being readmitted are 2.13 times greater for CHF patients than other patients in the study (see Note 2).

The effect of gender, another dichotomous independent variable, on readmission can be interpreted through the odds ratio: $e^{.44}$ or 1.55. Thus the odds of readmission for a female are one and one-half times the odds of readmission for a male. Note that this variable does not reach statistical significance when testing the beta coefficient; thus, the odd ratio of 1.55 is not considered large enough to be claimed significant. As Fleiss (1981) notes, values for odds ratios greater than or equal to 2.5 or 3.0 are generally taken to represent the lower limits of a strong association.

The coefficient of .06 on the continuous measure of functional dependency means that, on the average, the log odds for readmission increase by .06 for each unit increase in patient dependency level. For two patients with functional scores which differ by 18 points (one very independent with a score of 5 and one very dependent with a score of 23), the difference in log odds of readmission is .06(18) = 1.08; the associated odds ratio is $e^{1.08}$ which equals 2.94. Thus, a patient with a functional score of 23 has an odds of readmission that is about 2.9 the odds for a patient with a score of 5.

Finally, a very different approach to interpreting coefficients looks at the relationship between an independent variable and the dependent variable at a particular point along the curve. Although some statisticians criticize such attempts because it neglects the inherently interactive effects of the predictors on the probability (DeMaris, 1990), such interpretations are widely used (Teachman and Morgan, 1990). Through this approach, coefficients are translated directly into change in probability associated with incremental change in the independent variable. By taking the derivative of $P(Y = 1)$ with respect to X_1, one can see the rate of change in Y associated with a small change in X_1 (Aldrich & Nelson, 1984).

$$\frac{\blacktriangle \Pr(Y=1)}{\blacktriangle X_1} \dagger \ b_1 \ (P) \ (1-P)$$

This formula represents the change in the probability of being in category 1 (i.e., being readmitted) that is associated with a unit change in X_1, evaluated at the point at which the dependent variable takes on the value P. Thus, for every value of P (or every point on the axis representing the probability of being in category 1), the effect of the independent variable is different. The parameter estimate (b) remains constant in the equation but the values of (P) and (1–P) change and therefore the resulting product changes, showing that the relationship between the dependent variable and independent variable varies at points along the curve. The sign on the b coefficient always indicates the direction of the effect, but the magnitude of the effect varies with different values of P. Thus, the investigator must decide the particular value of P at which the relationship will be evaluated.

In selecting a value of P, usually a point is chosen on the curve which represents the actual probability of occurrence of the event in the population, and the impact of X_1 is evaluated at that point. For example, the readmission rate for the total sample is approximately 20%. Evaluated at that point of the curve (P = .20), a unit change in functional dependency is associated with a 1% change in probability of readmission ($.06 \times .20 \times .80 = .01$). One can also examine the effect of an independent variable at other probability levels of the dependent variable. The mid-point of the curve or the extremes may be of particular interest. In the readmission example, where the probability of readmission is .50, a unit change in functional status represents a 1.5% change in probability of readmission. However, where the probability of readmission is .10, a unit change in function status represents a .5% change in the probability of readmission (see Note 3 for calculations).

THE GOODNESS OF FIT OF THE MODEL

How well the model fits the data can be assessed through several different statistics, not all of which are yet commonly accepted in logistic regression. Since various computer packages produce different statistics, the manual for the specific program used should be consulted for information about the options among statistical tests available in that package.

In the SAS program, two model statistics are printed: the score statistic and the likelihood ratio chi-square statistic. Both are produced in similar ways and should be comparable in size. The likelihood ratio chi-square is the preferred statistic when convergence is obtained (Harrel, 1983). The likelihood ratio compares the likelihood function for the full model to the likelihood function if all coefficients except the intercept are 0. The resulting statistic follows a chi-square distribution when the null hypothesis is true. A chi-square table, using K-1 degrees of freedom, with K being the number of estimators in the model, is used to ascertain the probability level. In Table 1, the likelihood ratio statistic is labeled *-2 log L.R.* and equals 11.06 for the readmission model, a value with a probability of .0114 of occurring by chance. Thus, the overall model is statistically significant. The score statistic is similar: 10.97, with a probability of .0119.

SAS prints a statistic similar to the multiple correlation coefficient in OLS regression. It is sometimes referred to as the pseudo-R. The R takes on a value from -1 to +1, with a larger magnitude representing a better fitting model. R has a value of 0 if the model is a poor fit and a value of 1 if the model predicts perfectly (Harrel, 1983). Individual R statistics (partial R's) are computed for each independent variable in the model. They provide a measure of the contribution of each independent variable to predicting the dependent variable. As shown in Table 1, the R is equal to .119, indicating that the model does not fit the data very well. This information is also provided by the correlation coefficients at the bottom of the table. Four coefficients are produced, each of which provides some index of the rank correlation between the predicted probabilities and the observed values: C, Somer D, Gamma, Tau. The specific calculations differ (for example, in the method of dealing with pairs which tie on the predicted probability). In the example, the values of these statistics are small, indicating the relatively poor predictive ability of the model.

WHEN TO USE LOGISTIC REGRESSION

In the analyses of dichotomous dependent variables, social work researchers often use an ordinary least squares regression procedure and defend its use on several grounds, including its simplicity, robustness, relative economic computational methods, and straightforward interpretation (Cleary and Angel, 1984). Indeed, if the dependent variable has comparable numbers in each category, results are not substantially different from logistic procedures (Aldrich & Cnudde, 1975). However, the use of OLS with a binary dependent variable is technically incorrect because several assumptions are violated. Binary dependent variables are not normally distributed, the dependent variable and independent variables do not have a continuous linear relationship, and the error terms are not independent nor homoscedastic. Nerlove and Press (1973) argue that the estimators produced by OLS procedures are inefficient in that they do not have the smallest possible standard error and the estimated standard errors do not necessarily get closer to the true values as sample size increases. Also, the predicted values of Y will not be constrained between 0 and 1, which is inconsistent with the definition of probability. Aldrich and Nelson (1984) point out that OLS seriously mis-estimates the magnitude of the effects of independent variables and that standard inferential statistical tests are unjustified. The more unequally the dependent variable is distributed, the more inaccurate the OLS estimates will be. When the dependent variable is skewed beyond an 80-20 split, logistic parameters provide consistently better estimates.

Logistic regression is among a group of statistical techniques which are used in the analysis of dichotomous dependent variables. These include weighted least squares regression, probit analysis, and discriminant analysis. Discriminant analysis is perhaps the most familiar to social workers (see Cleary and Angel, 1984, and Aldrich and Nelson, 1984, for discussions of weighted least squares and probit analysis). The basic strategy of discriminant analysis is to form a linear combination of the independent variables and then to assign an observation to group 1 or group 2 based on the predicted value resulting from the equation (Kleinbaum, Kupper, and Muller, 1988). A linear function is estimated, and if the value of this function is above a certain cut-off, the observation is predicted to be in one category. The coefficients are linear transformations of the OLS regression coefficients, and they can be compared to assess their relative contribution to the discriminant function.

The purposes of discriminant analysis and logistic regression analysis are slightly different. Discriminant analysis is used to identify a set of predictors which best discriminates two groups of observations, with the goal being the assignment of observations to correct categories. Logistic regression is used to make inferences about the relationship of an independent and dependent variable, and the interpretation of the effect of the independent variable is straightforward.

Each procedure has its advantages. An advantage of discriminant analysis is that the coefficients can be found with a direct analytic solution and so computations are simpler than with logistic methods (Cleary and Angel, 1984). Also, when the sample size is small, discriminant analysis yields more efficient results than does logistic analysis. However, discriminant analysis is based on the assumptions of multivariate normality of the independent variables and equal covariance matrices. These assumptions are difficult to meet with small samples and when dependent variables are dichotomous (Lee, 1980). The advantage of logistic regression is that there are no such assumptions about the independent variables. In the case where these assumptions cannot be met, logistic regression is more appropriate than discriminant analysis (Press and Wilson, 1978). Another advantage of logistic analysis is that independent variables can also be dichotomous, a problematic situation in discriminant analysis. Finally, logistic regression can accommodate an extremely skewed distribution of the dependent variable, while discriminant analysis can not.

THE USE OF LOGISTIC REGRESSION IN THE SOCIAL WORK LITERATURE

The authors conducted a search of 7 major social work journals over the last 10 years to analyze the use of logistic regression by social work researchers. Journals were *Social Work, Social Work Research and Abstracts, Social Service*

Review, Journal of Social Service Research, Social Casework, Health and Social Work, and *Administration in Social Work.* A research assistant manually searched each article, looking for the terms "logistic," "log-odds," "odds ratio," and "log-linear" within the method, presentation of findings, and discussion sections. Given the difficulty of identifying a particular statistical analysis, the search may not be exhaustive. Ten articles were found to have been published in the ten-year period, as shown in Table 2.

The table shows the variety of important topics in social work which investigators measured dichotomously. It is interesting to note that five of the ten articles addressed aspects of service utilization. Similarly, three other articles analyzed factors associated with the occurrence of discrete events-pregnancy, discharge from a nursing home, and particular complications which plague discharge planning. Two articles address client satisfaction and income receipt-variables which lend themselves to continuous measurement. These authors report that problems with extremely limited distributions required categorization, hence the use of logistic regression (Morrow-Howell and Leon, 1987; Nichols-Casebolt, 1986). Thus social work researchers have used logistic regression when (1) binary dependent variables are substantively appropriate, and (2) the distribution of a continuous variable suggests the need to collapse to categories.

Many dependent variables of interest to social work are categorical, although as Kerlinger (1986) notes, categorical variables are "always quantifiable, or they are not variables." Stymied by difficulties in analyzing categorical variables and tempted by advances in statistical analyses for continuous dependent variables, researchers may attempt to substitute continuous measures for the phenomenon of interest best measured dichotomously. Yet as continuous measurements have continued to replace qualitative classifications, computer software for optimally analyzing qualitative data has become more widely available. Thus investigators need not substitute continuous measures with less direct appeal, nor need they rely on weaker methods of analysis when variables are measured dichotomously. Conversely of course, continuous measures should not be collapsed to a binary level when the result is an unnecessary loss of information. In sum, investigators should maintain appropriate correspondence between the research question of interest, the level of measurement of key variables, and the statistical analysis employed.

Studies in the social work literature reflect a variety of approaches for reporting and discussing the results of logistic analysis, as shown in Table 2. The table is organized to highlight three types of information which result from logistic analysis: tests of estimated coefficients, interpretation of those coefficients, and the goodness of the model. As discussed earlier in the paper, for each of these issues, the same information can be determined through alternative approaches.

For tests of coefficients, only one article presents MLE chi-square values. All others rely on t-tests but reflect wide variability in presentation. Some authors report values of the coefficients themselves, some report values of t-tests on the coefficients, some report probabilities associated with the t-values, and some report various combinations of these.

With respect to the interpretation of coefficients, half of the articles present information about direction of the relationship only. In the other articles, coefficients are interpreted further by presenting the magnitude of effects–either by calculating odds ratios or by presenting the change in probability associated with change in a given independent variable.

With respect to assessing the fit of the model, researchers have the widest range of options; however the appropriateness of various options seems subject to controversy. As Table 2 shows, social work researchers present model chi-squares, classification tables, sensitivity and specificity of classification, kappa statistics, likelihood ratio test statistics, pseudo R's, and fraction of concordant pairs, among other approaches.

The wide variation in approach to reporting and interpreting findings reflects, in part, the state of art regarding logistic regression. Various computer packages use alternative approaches to conveying basically the same information, and to date there seems to be no consensus about what is "right." Other variations in approach to interpreting regression analysis may be discipline related. For example, economists and epidemiologists appear to approach the interpretation of coefficients differently. Epidemiologists tend to use odds ratios, while economists more often report changes in probability. Social work research may be particularly subject to heterogeneity in approach because social work has traditionally borrowed its methodology from various social sciences.

This wide diversity in reporting is not without negative consequences. Indeed it may be a prime contributor to confusion about logistic regression among both investigators and consumers of research. Researchers who use logistic regression may be uncertain about how to report their findings and attempts to find a "model" in the social work literature may be futile, given the variation reflected in Table 2. However, the lack of consensus about the "right" way to present findings does not excuse investigators from fully reporting and interpreting their findings.

Complete presentation of logistic regression usually requires that the investigator present information regarding the statistical significance of coefficients and interpret at least the direction of the relationship. In addition, computing the magnitude of the relationship is as central to the interpretation of the results as in OLS regression (Alba, 1987). This paper shows the feasibility and usefulness of interpreting the coefficients and encourages social work researchers to provide fuller interpretations. Finally, although the aim of a study may not be prediction or model building, some indication of the goodness of the model is appropriate.

Logistic regression is infrequently used in the social work literature, as reflected in the fact that our search identified only 10 articles in 10 years. However, as shown here, it is the most appropriate technique for the analysis of many dependent variables of interest to social work researchers.

TABLE 2

LOGISTIC REGRESSION IN SOCIAL WORK JOURNALS

AUTHOR	JOURNAL	DEPENDENT VARIABLE	TEST OF COEFFICIENTS	INTERPRETATIONS OF COEFFICIENTS	GOODNESS OF MODEL
Dove, Schneider & Gitelson, 1985	SW	Need for social work services versus no need	Not presented	Magnitude: Adjusted odds ratio presented in table but not discussed in text	Not presented
Judge & Smith, 1983	SSR	Agency purchase of service versus direct provision	t-values reported with significance noted	Direction of relationship discussed in text	Likelihood ratio test statistic reported with significance noted
Keefe, 1983	SSR	Pregnancy	t-values reported, significance not noted	Direction & Magnitude: change in probability associated with unit change in independent variable.	Not presented
Morrow-Howell Clark, Miller, 1987	Health & SW	Nursing home discharge	(a) probability level reported but no t-value presented (b) D statistic (partial r)	Direction & Magnitude: Change in probability associated with unit change in independent variable	Classification table; sensitivity, specificity, and Kappa.
Morrow-Howell, & Leon, 1987	JSSR	Receipt of any money from family versus no receipt	(a) probability level reported but no t-value presented (b) partial r	Direction of relationship discussed in text	Model R; Score statistic; Fraction of Concordant Pairs and Rank Correlation

TABLE 2 CONTINUED

AUTHOR	JOURNAL	DEPENDENT VARIABLE	TEST OF COEFFICIENTS	INTERPRETATIONS OF COEFFICIENTS	GOODNESS OF MODEL
Neighbors & Taylor, 1985	SSR	Use of social services	Statistical significant relationship described in text but no values reported	Direction and Magnitude: Odds ratio presented and interpreted	Model X2 and Significance
Nichols-Casebolt 1986	SSR	Satisfied of welfare recipients vs not satisfied	t-values reported with significance noted	Direction of relationship discussed in text	Model significance reported but no model x^2 presented
Proctor & Morrow-Howell, 1990	Health & SW	Occurance of Complicatons in discharge planning	MLE x^2 values and probability levels reported	Direction of relationship discussed in text	Pseudo R and Significance levels reported
Sosin, 1987	SWRA	Type of social problems covered by private agencies	(a) significant coefficients noted based on unreported t-tests; and (b) significance of change in model chi-square	Directions of relationship sign of coefficient discussed in text.	Model x^2 and significance
Sosin, 1985	SSR	Type of social problems covered by private agencies	(a)statistically significant coefficient values presented; and (b) change in model x^2 statistic and significance noted	Direction of relationship discussed in text	Not presented

101

NOTES

1. $Y = -2.76 + .76 (X_1) + .06 (X_2) + .44 (X_3)$

   $\hat{Y} = -2.76 + .76 (1) + .06 (8) + .44 (1)$

   $\hat{Y} = -1.08$ [the log odds of readmission]

   $e^{-1.08} = .339$ [the odds of being readmitted]

   $Pr (Y = 1) = 1/[1 + e^{-(-1.08)}]$

   $= \dfrac{1}{1 + 2.9446}$

   $= .25$ [the probability of being readmitted]

2. To understand this odds ratio more completely, one could calculate the probability of readmission for a female patient with CHF and a functional dependency score of 8, which is .25 as noted above; then a similar calculation could be made on a female patient with the same level of dependency at discharge but with a non-CHF diagnosis. The probability of readmission for this patient is .14. There is an 11 percent difference in probability. Converting these probabilities to odds (.25 probability equals the odds of .34; .14 probability equals the odds of .16) and comparing them by division yields the odds ratio of .34/.16 or 2.13.

3. $\dfrac{\blacktriangle Prob\ (Y=1)}{\blacktriangle X_1} = b (P)(1-P)$ where $P = .50$

   $= .06 (.50)(1-.50)$

   $= .015$

   $\dfrac{\blacktriangle Prob\ (Y=1)}{\blacktriangle X_1} = b(P)(1-p)$ where $P = .10$

   $= .06 (.10)(1-.10)$

   $= .005$

REFERENCES

Alba, R. (1987). Interpreting the parameters of log-linear models. *Sociological Methods and Research*, 16(1), 45-77.

Aldrich, J. & Cnudde, C. (1975). Probing the bounds of conventional wisdom: A comparison of regression, probit, and discriminant analysis. *American Journal of Political Science*, 19(3), 571-608.

Aldrich, J. & Nelson, F. (1984). *Linear probability, logit, and probit Models*. Beverly Hills: Sage Publications.

Cleary, P. & Angel, R. (1984). The analysis of relationships involving dichotomous dependent variables. *Journal of Health & Social Behavior*, 25(3), 334-348.

Cox, D. R. (1977). *The analysis of binary data*. London: Methuen.

DeMaris, (1990). Interpreting logistic regression results: A critical commentary. *Journal of Marriage and the Family*, 52, 271-276.

Dove, H.G., Schneider, K.C., & Gitelson, David A. (1985). Identifying patients who need social work services: An interdisciplinary analysis. *Social Work*, 30(3), 214-218.

Engelman, L. (1983). Stepwise logistic regression. *BMDP Statistical Software*. Berkeley: University of California Press, pp. 330-344.

Everitt, B. S. (1977). *The analysis of contingency tables.* New York: Halsted Press.

Fleiss, J. (1981). *Statistical methods for rates and proportions.* New York: John Wiley.

Harrel, F. (1983). The logist procedure. *SUGI Supplemental Library User's Guide*. Cary, North Carolina: SAS Institute, pp. 181-202.

Judge, K. & Smith, J. (1983). Purchase of service in England. *Social Service Review*, 57(2), 209-233.

Keefe, D.E. (1983). Governor Reagan, welfare reform, and AFDC fertility. *Social Service Review*, 57(2), 234-253.

Kerlinger, F. (1986). *Foundations of behavioral research.* New York: CBS College Publishing.

Kleinbaum, D., Kupper, L., & Muller, K. (1988). *Applied regression analysis and other multivariable methods*. Boston: PWS-Kent Publishing.

Knoke, D. & Burke, P. (1980). *Log-linear models*. Beverly Hills: Sage Publications.

Lee, E. (1980). *Statistical methods for survival data analysis.* Belmont, CA: Wadsworth.

Morgan, S. & Teachman, J. (1988). Logistic regression: Descriptions, examples, and comparisons. *Journal of Marriage and the Family*, 50, 271-277.

Morrow-Howell, N. & Leon, J. (1987). The Family as an Income Source for the Older Adult. *Journal of Social Service Research*, 11(1), 1-16.

Morrow-Howell, N., Clark, W. F., & Miller, L. S. (1987). Multipurpose senior services program deinstitutionalization screen. *Health and Social Work*, 12(3), 197-204.

Neighbors, H. W., & Taylor, R. (1985). The Use of Social Service Agencies by Black Americans. *Social Service Review*, 59(2), 258-268.

Nerlove, M. & Press, S.J. (1973). *Univariate and multivariate log-linear and logistic models*. Santa Monica, CA: Rand Corporation.

Nichols-Casebolt, A. (1986). The Psychological Effects of Income Testing Income-Support Benefits. *Social Service Review*, 60(2), 287-302.

Press, S.J. & Wilson, T.P. (1978). Choosing between logistic regression and discriminant analysis. *Journal of the American Statistical Association*, 73, 699-705.

Proctor, E. K. and Morrow-Howell, N. (1990). Complications in discharge planning with Medicare patients. *Health and Social Work*, 15(1), 45-54.

Sosin, M. (1985). Social problems covered by private agencies: An application of niche theory. *Social Service Review*, 59(1), 75-94.
Sosin, M. (1987). Private social agencies: auspices, sources of funds, and problems covered. *Social Work Research and Abstract*, 23(2), 21-27.
Teachman, J. & Morgan, S. (1990). A brief response to DeMaris. *Journal of Marriage and the Family*, 52, 276.
Walsh, A. (1987). Teaching understanding and interpretation of logit regression. *Teaching Sociology*, 15(2), 178-183.

Loglinear Analysis in Social Work Research

Terri Combs-Orme

SUMMARY. Loglinear analysis is a method of statistical analysis that is used when all the variables of interest are categorical. The method has had wide use in the social sciences, but has not been used extensively in social work research. Loglinear analysis has several advantages over less appropriate methods that tend to be used frequently in social work research. Among the most important of those advantages is the capability of accounting for multicollinearity among variables; multiple bivariate tests cannot detect such relationships and may thus produce distorted and misleading results. This article explains the appropriate uses of loglinear analysis, describes briefly the calculations involved, and finally illustrates applications of the method.

In social work research both the independent and the dependent variables are frequently categorical or nominal variables. For example, one may ask whether abused children are more likely to be placed in foster care than neglected children, whether female homeless clients find it more difficult to obtain shelter than males, etc.

Loglinear analysis (Goodman, 1971, 1972) is a statistical method that is appropriate for categorical independent and dependent variables that has had wide application in related professional literature (e.g., Aneshensel, 1983;

Terri Combs-Orme is Assistant Professor in the Department of Maternal and Child Health, School of Hygiene and Public Health, Johns Hopkins University. She earned her PhD at Washington University in St. Louis. Her current research concerns health care access and use by disadvantaged mothers and children. She is working on projects concerning prenatal care for drug-using women; prenatal care for low-income rural and Hispanic women in New Mexico; and completing a paper on predictors of birthweight using the National Natality Survey. Related article: Combs-Orme, T., Helzer, J., and Miller, R. (1987-88). The application of labeling theory to alcoholism. *Journal of Social Service Research*, *11* (2/3), 73-91.

The author wishes to express gratitude to John G. Orme, Joe Crymes, and Rebecca Hegar for valuable comments on an earlier draft of this manuscript.

© 1992 by The Haworth Press, Inc. All rights reserved.

Fleiss, Williams, & Dubro, 1986), but relatively infrequent use in social work research. This paper examines loglinear analysis and its utility for social work researchers, using illustrations from social work research. The first section describes research problems that are appropriate for the use of loglinear analysis, with particular attention to advantages over other typically used statistical methods. The second section describes briefly the calculations for loglinear analysis, and the various types of models. The third section discusses the testing of models, while the final section considers a number of important issues for the appropriate application of loglinear analysis.

WHEN TO USE LOGLINEAR ANALYSIS

Loglinear analysis is appropriate when all study variables, including independent and dependent variables, are categorical. In cases where the dependent variable is dichotomous and the independent variables are a mixture of continuous and categorical, logistic regression is a more appropriate method. (See Morrow-Howell & Proctor, this issue.) Extensions of loglinear analysis recently have been developed for ordinal data as well (Norusis, 1988; Wickens, 1989). These extensions are similar to the general loglinear model, with added terms to express the ordinal nature of the variables.

In a typical study that is appropriate for loglinear analysis, Combs-Orme, Helzer, and Miller (1987/88) wished to determine the effects of being labeled "alcoholic" by various persons (self, family, and others) on subsequent drinking patterns, testing the theory that being labeled as a deviant results in subsequent deviant behavior. In order to address this question, it was necessary to account for a number of other interrelated factors that are associated with drinking patterns, including race and severity of life-problems related to drinking. For example, before one could conclude that being labeled as an "alcoholic" by one's family results in alcoholic drinking patterns, it would be necessary to account for the effects of the severity of symptoms on the label itself. This is because persons with more symptoms would be more likely to be labeled an alcoholic, and also more likely to have problems later on.

Social work researchers often have analyzed similar categorical data by performing multiple bivariate tests, e.g., Chi-square analyses of contingency tables to examine separately the effects of each independent variable on the outcome variable. The use of multiple contingency tables has been a traditional method of searching for various types of relationships among variables, including interactions and spurious relationships (Rosenberg, 1968). However, such an approach is likely to obscure or distort true relationships as a result of failing to take the associations among the independent variables into account, and it also may result in inflated Type I error rates. Moreover, Fienberg (1981) notes that this approach ignores the possibility of higher order interactions among the variables. For example, in the alcoholic labeling study discussed above (Combs-Orme et al., 1987/88), a simple contingency table approach would have resulted in the erroneous conclusion that gender, race, and alcoholic labels from any source were significantly related to outcomes, when in fact only the seriousness of alcohol problems and gender were related to drinking outcomes.

Unfortunately the social work literature is replete with examples of this error. In one example of such an error, Jenkins, Diamond, Flanzraich, Gibson, Hendricks, and Marshood (1983) studied over 300,000 children in foster care to determine whether ethnicity affects a number of outcome variables including legal status, type of placement, location of placement, and length of time in foster care. Using at least six Chi-square tests, the authors reported significant effects for ethnicity on legal status, type of placement, location of placement, and length of time in care. In the only reported analyses where the minority status was broken out into Black, American Indian, Asian, and Hispanic groups, as opposed to a majority/minority dichotomy, the authors reported significant differences among the ethnic groups for type of placement and length of care.

This study illustrates well the inadequacy of bivariate tests. Given the high likelihood that correlated independent variables may have produced spurious relationships, a more complex examination of the relationships among all the independent variables would be appropriate. Indeed, loglinear analysis provides the same information as multiple contingency table analysis, but is able to provide important additional information. For example, it is possible that only one of the independent variables is causally related to the outcomes, but that the inter-correlations among the independent variables resulted in spurious relationships with others. This possibility can only be addressed if all variables are tested simultaneously. The large sample in this study would have permitted such simultaneous testing without the danger of inadequate cell sizes.

In the face of such difficulties, many researchers might turn to multiple regression using dummy variables, even though the dichotomous nature of these variables constitutes a violation of the assumptions of multiple regression (Cohen & Cohen, 1983). Although multiple regression is a robust method, this situation, and in particular the dichotomous dependent variable, constitutes a serious enough violation of the normality assumption as to present insurmountable problems (Cleary & Angel, 1984). Loglinear analysis is clearly the statistical method of choice in these situations.

Loglinear analysis can follow either of two models: the general loglinear model, or the special case of logit analysis. The general model examines relationships among several response variables and assumes no dependent variable. It might be used when the researcher is not interested in what causes a specific phenomenon, but rather how several factors such as race, gender, and self-esteem are related to each other. Logit analysis, on the other hand, is a special sub-class of loglinear analysis that examines the effects of several independent variables on a dependent (or response) variable.

Operations of the two models are similar when the response variable is dichotomous and the results concerning the response variable are the same, with the exception that loglinear models, unlike logit models, must include terms for the relationships among all the independent variables. As a result, compared to the general loglinear model, the corresponding logit model for the same data contains fewer terms (Wickens, 1989, pp. 181-186).

COMPUTATION OF THE LOGLINEAR MODEL

Extensive statistical training is not necessary to use loglinear appropriately, but a basic understanding of several fundamental issues is needed. It is helpful to refer to the familiar two-way Chi-square test, beginning with the underlying assumptions which also apply to loglinear analysis (Hays, 1988). In brief, the assumptions are that data are independent observations derived from multinomial sampling, with larger samples resulting in a closer approximation to the Chi-square distribution. Although the Chi-square test is relatively robust, gross violations call results into question.

In the simplest use of loglinear, as in the Chi-square test, one may wish to test whether two variables in a cross-classification table are related. In such a test, expected frequencies are computed for each cell of the table and compared to the observed frequencies. The expected frequencies are derived by simply multiplying the row totals by the column totals, and dividing by the total number of observations. If the two variables are unrelated, the expected and observed frequencies will be very close.

The first step of a loglinear analysis is much the same as the Chi-square test. For example, the first step of analysis in the Combs-Orme et al. (1987/88) study was to test for marginal and partial associations in the observed frequencies (also called the full "saturated" model; this term is defined and discussed below). This test of the marginal associations corresponds exactly to simple Chi-square tests.

Table 1 demonstrates numerous significant marginal associations, as shown in the second column of the table. Indeed, only race (not shown in the table) was not significantly associated with other independent variables on the marginal tests, as the significant interactions show. The smaller values of the partial associations for each effect show that the relationship is reduced after accounting for the effects of other variables.

The null hypothesis of no relationship in a two-way table essentially means that the percentages for each variable are the same across the levels of the other variable.[1] For example, race was not significant in the Combs-Orme et al. (1987/88) study because Blacks and whites were equally likely to have very serious alcohol problems, to be labeled as "alcoholic" by each source, and to have poor drinking outcomes. Thus race was not related to any other variable, and it was not included in further analyses.

Unrelatedness thus implies a situation wherein the expected frequencies can be determined by the total number of cases and the marginal (row and column) totals, with the following model:

Formula 1:
Expected frequency = (Row probability × Column probability) × N

The term "loglinear" derives from the logarithmic transformation, which results in a linear formula. Formula 2, below, is the logarithmic transformation of Formula 1. The skeptical reader can verify the relationship between the two formulas by following Wickens's (1989) example (p. 35). As the reader may recall, a transformation to natural logarithms (base e = 2.71828) changes products to sums and powers to products.

Formula 2:
Log of expected frequency = constant + (row term) + (column term)

Formulas 1 and 2 are models of independence under the null hypothesis. It is easy to extend the formula to describe association between the two variables by adding a term:

Formula 3:
Log of expected frequency = constant + row term + column term + association

Most of the major texts and the computer programs use scientific notation for such formulas. Formula 4, as written below according to the notation used in SPSS, for example, is identical to Formula 3.

Formula 4:
$$\ln F_m = \mu + \lambda_i^H + \lambda_j^S + \lambda_{ij}^{HS}$$

In this notation, the constant, μ, is the average value of all the cells of the table. The row, column, and association terms are written as lambdas (λ), which act to increase (for values above 1.0) or decrease (for values below 1.0) the logged probabilities of the row and column effects. (The lambda term is similar to an unstandardized regression coefficient, and is computed by taking the average log of the frequencies in a particular category, minus the grand mean.) The association term adjusts for the relationship between the row and column variables. (There is no association term in the formula for independence, because it is zero.) Thus the transformation results in a linear equation, which is analogous to linear regression, in that each variable can be expressed as a constant, plus terms representing relationships to other variables.

Table 1

Significant Likelihood Ratio Associations In the Saturated Model

Effect	Partial Association	Marginal Association	Odds Ratio (Marginal Association)	
Self X Family	24.50	51.57		6.5
Outside X Family	13.32	36.20		4.6
Outside X Self	4.29	26.59		3.6
Severity X Self	18.99	47.23		4.6
Severity X Outside	12.63	36.55		4.5
Gender X Outcome	4.10	8.53		0.3
Severity X Outcome	11.45	26.70		9.6
Gender X Self	0.17	3.86		0.6
Gender X Family	0.90	4.69		0.6
Gender X Severity	2.70	8.31		0.5
Severity X Family	2.77	28.18		3.7
Self X Outcome	2.17	15.08		4.9
Outside X Outcome	0.89	9.53		3.1
Family X Outcome	1.40	11.95		3.6
Gender X Outside X Outcome 5.40		2.18	Men	1.7
			Women	5.3
			M-H	2.9
Gender X Severity X Family 5.51		1.91	Men	4.8
			Women	1.9
			M-H	3.4

From Combs-Orme, Helzer, & Miller, 1987/88.

p < .001
p < .05
p < .01

It is the application to multi-way tables that illustrates most clearly the advantages of loglinear analysis. That is, the logarithmic formula provides a method of expressing the expected frequency for each cell as a combination of a constant and a series of terms expressing relationships with the other variables, and simultaneously comparing the expected and observed values for every cell in the table. It was not possible to perform such simultaneous tests with large contingency tables before the availability of high-speed computers. The iterative method that is used by the computer to compute these expected values is the Maximum Likelihood Estimate (MLE) method, which is well explained for the curious reader by Wickens (1989, pp. 107-112) and by Fienberg (1981, pp. 37-40). For others, it is only important to know that the MLE method is an iterative process that provides the most efficient estimates of the expected frequencies with the lowest standard errors.

In loglinear analysis then, the logs of expected frequencies (based on the hypothesis of independence, or based upon some other hypothesized relationship among the variables) are compared to the logs of the observed frequencies, using the logged odds ratio. Before the method of comparing the observed and expected values is discussed, an understanding of the odds ratio may be helpful.

The Odds Ratio

An understanding of the odds ratio is important to loglinear analysis, because the method actually uses the log odds as the dependent variable, rather than the frequencies. It is useful to discuss the odds ratio from the base of an example.

The odds ratio (also called the "cross-product ratio") is based on the "odds." The odds of an event is a simple ratio of the probability of its occurrence, divided by the probability of its not occurring. For example, in the United States 5.6 percent of white women deliver infants who are low birthweight, that is less than approximately 5 1/2 pounds at birth (Hughes, Johnson, Rosenbaum, Simons, & Butler, 1987). Thus the probability of a LBW for a white birth is slightly over 5 percent. The odds of a low birthweight infant for a white mother (.056/1-.056) are relatively low: 5.93 percent or about 1 in 17.

The odds ratio is a measure of the relative odds of some outcome for one group based on some characteristic or exposure to some risk factor, compared to the odds for another group. Using the above example, in contrast to white infants, the probability of LBW for African-American babies is about .124 (12.4 percent) (Hughes et al., 1987). An African-American mother's odds of a LBW are thus .124/.876, which is equal to 14.16 percent or about 1 in 7. The odds ratio is a measure of the ratio of the two odds. Thus an African-American mother's risk compared to that for her white counterpart is 1 in 7 compared to 1 in 17, or 2.4. Therefore, an African-American mother is over twice as likely as a white mother to give birth to a baby who is too small at birth.

Like other measures of association such as Phi or Yule's Q, the odds ratio is important because it is unaffected by sample size. Larger samples yield larger Chi-square values solely because of the sample size, but the odds ratio is affected only by the association between the variables.

The odds ratio is often called the "cross-product ratio" because it may be derived as follows. Using data presented in Table 2, the ratio of the major diagonal (23 × 35) to the minor diagonal (77 × 7), is computed and equals 1.5.

In this example, it would be concluded that African-American mothers are 1.5 times as likely (or 50 percent more likely) to deliver LBW babies as white mothers.

The race variable would have no effect in this example if the odds of the outcome were the same for each group, and the Odds Ratio would equal 1. The cells of a two-way table are, of course, positioned arbitrarily. Therefore, it is usually most meaningful to position them so that the resulting odds ratio is one or greater, but this is not necessary. The rows and columns may be reversed and the Odds Ratio expressed as a fraction. The greater the Odds Ratio, the stronger is the association between the two variables. For more information on the Odds Ratio, the reader should see Fleiss (1981).

Table 2

Models Tested In Predicting Outcome

Model	df	Likelihood Ratio Statistic	P
1. (I),(M)	62	84.78	.03
2. (I),(PM),(SM)	87	86.04	.51
3. (I),(GM),(PM)	87	86.27	.50
4. (I),(PM),(FM)	87	86.53	.49
5. (I),(PM),(OM)	87	88.67	.43
6. (I),(GFM)	86	85.73	.49
7. (I),(PSM)	86	83.48	.56
8. (I),(PFM)	86	86.45	.47
9. (I),(PM),(GM),(SM)	86	81.35	.62
10. (I),(PM),(GM),(OM)	86	83.55	.55
11. (I),(PM),(GM),(FM)	86	81.71	.61
12. (I),(PM),(GM),(FM),(OM)	85	80.50	.62
13. (I),(PM),(GM),(OM),(SM)	85	79.62	.64

I = All possible interactions of independent variables
M = Drinking status at followup (moderate vs. nonmoderate)
P = Lifetime number of drinking problems
G = Gender
S = Alcoholic self-label
F = Alcoholic label by family
O = Alcoholic label by outsiders

Hierarchical models imply the inclusion of all constituents lower-order terms when higher order effects are included, e.g. "MG" implies "M" and "G."

From Combs-Orme, Helzer, & Miller, 1987/88.

TESTING MODELS

Basic Models

The researcher's ultimate purpose in testing models is to build a model containing the important variables that describe his or her data as well as possible. There are a number of steps that are performed to that end, but first it is important to understand the most fundamental models. One, the model of independence, was discussed above and expressed in Formulas 1 and 2. This model simply assumes that there are no relationships among the variables in the observed frequencies.

Another important model is the "saturated model," also mentioned above. Quite simply, the saturated model is the full representation of the data, including all possible main effects and interaction parameters. Although it represents the data perfectly (the expected and observed frequencies are identical), the saturated model has no practical usefulness because it contains the same number of terms as the table has cells. As more parsimonious models are specified by dropping terms from the model (that is, setting some parameters to zero), additional degrees of freedom are gained for testing the fit of those models.

Because the saturated model is a full representation of the data, all other, more parsimonious, models are subsets of the saturated model and may be compared to it. Thus in the search for the best representation of his or her data, the researcher compares various more parsimonious models to see which best represents the data.

Most methods of loglinear analysis require that in order to be compared to each other, models must be hierarchical; that is, one must be "nested" within the other. Two models are hierarchical if one is a subset of the other, that is if all of the factors of the simpler model are also part of the higher model. Higher order effects automatically imply all lower-order effects, so that if a model contains a three-way factor [ABC], it is implied that it also includes effects, [A], [B], and [C]; and all possible two-way effects, [AB], [BC], and [AC].

For example, an important finding of the Combs-Orme et al. (1987/88) study was that the combination of gender, severity of problems, and a label of "alcoholic" predicted outcomes well. This is demonstrated in Table 3, in models 9, 10, and 11. Inspection of the models shows that the three models have remarkably similar L^2 values, and that each is better than the fit of the simpler models 2 through 5. However, adding a second label from another source to those models did not improve appreciably the fit of any of those three models, as is shown in models 12 and 13.

Comparing Two Models

The comparison of two different models is performed using either the Pearson's Chi-square statistic or the Likelihood Ratio Test (L^2). L^2, called G^2 by some authors, is very similar to the Pearson's Chi-Square, and is used by some researchers because of its familiarity.

Table 3
Fabricated Data: Race and Birthweight

	Birthweight		
	Low	Normal	
Maternal Race Black	23	77	100
Maternal Race White	7	35	42
	30	112	142

Formula 5:
$$L^2 = 2 \times \text{(Sum of observed frequencies)} \times \left[\text{Log} \frac{\text{(Sum observed frequencies)}}{\text{(Sum expected frequencies)}}\right]$$

Some disagreement exists regarding which statistic is preferable, and there is merit to each side. In most cases the values are very close and likely to lead to the same conclusions. However, a major advantage of L^2 is that it can be partitioned, permitting the comparison of the adequacy of fit of models. (This process is explained and illustrated in detail below.)

Whether the Pearson's Chi-square test or the L^2 test is used, the value is compared to the Chi-square distribution with the appropriate degrees of freedom (equal to the number of cells in the table, minus the number of set parameters). Larger values, relative to the degrees of freedom, indicate a poor fit of the model to the data.

If the researcher is testing the model of independence, a statistically significant Chi-square indicates that the null hypothesis of no relationship is rejected and it is concluded that the variables are associated. The first model tested in the Combs-Orme et al. (1987/88) study (Table 3) is the model of independence. The L^2 value of 84.78 with 62 degrees of freedom was significant at the .03 level. This indicates that the model of independence does not fit the data. Therefore, that model is rejected and other models are then tested.

When the researcher is testing a model, a significant Chi-square indicates a poor fit and the researcher proceeds to reformulate the model. Thus, unlike other types of analysis, when the researcher is testing the fit of a model using loglinear analysis, he or she is not seeking a significant Chi-square value, but a non-significant one. This is because a non-significant Chi-square value indicates that there is no significant difference between the frequencies generated by the hypothesized model and the observed frequencies.

Partitioning. Partitioning consists of dividing the L^2 value into parts, permitting the comparison of the adequacy of fit of hierarchical models. That is, it is possible to use the change in L^2 when a term is added to a model to determine the improvement in fit of the model attributable to the new term.

There are two steps to using partitioning to compare the fit of two models. In the first step, one compares the L^2 and significance levels of the two models. Of course, a model with a statistically significant L^2 clearly does not fit the data and may be rejected, as in Table 3 the model of independence (Model 1) was rejected. For models that are not rejected, one may subtract the L^2 of one model from that of the other model and compare the remainder to the Chi-square distribution (using the difference in degrees of freedom between the two models). When the remainder is significant, it indicates that the new model provides a significant improvement in fit over the previous model. The reader should note that for this comparison of models, a significant L^2 indicates a significant improvement in fit. Thus, in the Combs-Orme et al. (1987/88) study, Model 11 was compared to Model 12 by subtracting 80.50 from 81.71. The difference (1.21) is not significant with 1 degree of freedom; Model 12 does not provide a significantly improved fit over Model 11.

The selection of a model using partitioning is not as simple as it might appear. First of all, comparisons are only appropriate between hierarchical (or "nested") models where one model is a subset of the other. For example, one may compare Models 11 and 12 in Table 3, but not Models 11 and 13, because neither is a subset of the other. Second, the selection of the most appropriate model is not always a simple matter of choosing the model with the largest "p" value. Even given a nonsignificant model and a statistically significant improvement of that model over the alternative, one may select a model based on parsimony and simplicity of interpretation, or upon substantive knowledge or theory. In particular, the addition of higher order terms presents difficulties in substantive interpretation.

Brown's study (1983) of Black adolescent parents is a good illustration of partitioning.[2] (See Table 4.) Brown was interested in the prediction of how young people perceived their relationship following an unplanned pregnancy. The dependent variable, the respondents' current perceptions of their relationship (designated "C"), was coded as "love" or "not love."

Brown tested models using independent variables of perception of the relationship before pregnancy ("love" vs. "not love") and the sex of the respondent ("S"). Table 4 demonstrates the proposed models, which were based on theory and previous research. By convention, variables within the same parentheses or braces are hypothesized to be associated, and those in separate parentheses are hypothesized to be independent. Thus, Model 1 in Table 4 shows that the perceptions of the relationship before pregnancy and the sex of the respondent are related, but that is neither related to the current perceptions of the relationship. Interactions are shown as combinations of the two variables, such as "AB" for an interaction between "A" and "B."

Testing began with the simplest model, hypothesizing in Model 1 that no relationship existed between the current perceptions of the relationship and

Table 4

Example of Hierarchical Model Testing

Model	Marginals Fitted	L	df	P
1	(BS) (C)	15.73	3	.001
2	(BS) (CB)	1.79	2	.409
3	(BS) (CS)	14.50	2	.001
4	(BS) (CS) (CS)	1.57	1	.209

B = Perception of relationship before pregnancy

S = Sex of respondent

C = Current perception of relationship

From Brown, 1983, p. 30

either gender or prior perceptions. All models assumed a relationship between gender and prior perceptions. A test of Model 1 resulted in an L^2 of 15.73 (df 3), which is highly significant, and indicates a poor fit.

The next step to finding a model with a better fit is a comparison of Model 1 to a hierarchical model. Both Model 2 and Model 3 fit this criterion and may be compared to Model 1. The two models should not be compared directly to each other, because one is not a subset of the other. Model 3, which hypothesizes a relationship between gender and current perceptions, is significant, indicating a poor fit, so it is rejected. Model 2, which hypothesizes a relationship between prior and current perceptions, fits well. Moreover, subtracting the smaller L^2 and degrees of freedom results in an L^2 (df 1) that indicates a significant improvement in fit. Model 2 appears to be a good choice.

As is common, however, Brown performed one more test of a hierarchical model of Model 3 to determine if the fit to the data could be improved further. The new model hypothesized an association between current perceptions and the respondent's sex. The resulting L^2 was not significant, indicating a reasonable fit, but it resulted in a nonsignificant improvement in fit over Model 2. Moreover, the addition of this term results in a loss of parsimony. Model 2 is thus preferred over Model 3 and was selected by the author as the most reasonable model to describe the data.

Brown's (1983) approach illustrates how one may begin with a hypothesized model to describe one's data based on previous research, and then proceed by adding or deleting terms to determine whether the fit can be improved. In cases where there is an inadequate foundation for hypothesizing a model, one might begin with the saturated model and proceed to delete terms to see how fit is affected. However, such "fishing" is discouraged because it is likely to capitalize on chance and this "strategy" becomes increasingly difficult as the number of variables involved increases (Agresti, 1990). In either case, it should be emphasized again that comparisons can be made only between hierarchical models.

Model construction might also take a path analysis-type approach, just as is common with linear multiple regression (Wickens, 1989; Agresti, 1990). That is, in some cases a researcher might hypothesize a series of causal relationships among variables, placing his or her variables in temporal, causal sequence. For example, the Combs-Orme et al. (1987/88) study used labeling theory to hypothesize that a label of "alcoholic" from family and others resulted first in an individual internalizing that label, and subsequently in the individual beginning to drink defiantly in response to the self-label. Temporal sequencing was necessary for support of the labeling theory. The path analysis approach is appealing because it requires the researcher to start from a base of knowledge about the subject, rather than capitalizing upon findings that may be due to chance and that may be difficult to interpret.

Of course in many cases there is inadequate information to posit such causal models. In such cases Agresti (1990) offers another approach whereby the researcher may narrow the range of potential models by testing first the model with only single-factor terms, then those with both single and two-factor terms, and so on. This method will provide information on the complexity of relationships among the variables.

Parameter Estimates

Just as in linear regression, model parameters indicate the strength and direction of associations between variables. However, in loglinear analysis a term is produced for each level of the categorical variables. Researchers report effect sizes using various parameters and each must be interpreted slightly differently. The use of different parameters merely reflects personal taste because the substantive conclusions are not different. It is nonetheless important for the reader to be clear on which parameter is being used.

A positive lambda indicates that the average number of cases in that category is larger than the overall average, and a negative indicates the converse. In interpretation, the sign of lambda indicates the direction of the effect, and the magnitude indicates how strongly the variables are associated. Since the natural log of 1.00 is zero, a lambda of zero in a model indicates no effect for that factor, just as in linear regression a variable with no effect has a slope of zero (Knoke & Burke, 1980).

Most computer programs also display the Standard Error (SE) of lambda, and the Z-score, which is simply lambda divided by its SE. The Z-score is interpreted as are other Z-scores; a value of 1.96 or above is considered significant at the .05 level. Some authors refer to the standardized lambda as τ or "tau," as did Combs-Orme et al. in Table 5.

The confidence intervals (CI) for lambda (λ) may be constructed in the usual manner:

Formula 6:
CI (λ) = (λ) +- (1.96) (SEλ)

As is usually the case with confidence intervals, if the CI does not include zero, one can reject the hypothesis that the population value is zero.

There are a number of other parameters that are produced by some computer packages and used by some authors. As with other methods, it is often useful to examine the differences between the expected and observed frequencies, the residuals. If the model fits the data well, the standardized residuals (the residuals, divided by their Standard Errors) are approximately normally distributed with a mean of zero and a standard deviation of one. Thus, standardized residuals greater than 1.96 (or less than -1.96) may be interpreted as statistically significant. A plot of the residuals may be useful when patterns suggest relationships to be added to a model.

Because multiplicative parameters are more common (readers are more accustomed to them) and more conceptually meaningful (as in the ease of interpretation of the odds ratio, for example), some authors also may present multiplicative parameter estimates such as Beta. A Beta of less than one indicates a negative association between the first level of an independent variable and the first level of the dependent variable.

As shown in Table 5, Combs-Orme et al. present effect sizes for several models with similar fit to their data. For example, taking into account the coding for the variables shown in the table, effect sizes for the model including gender and outcome show that: (1) males who were labeled by any source were less likely (Beta of less than 1) than females to be drinking moderately; and (2) this effect was statistically significant (Tau of over 1.96); and (3) the effects of the three types of labels on outcome were remarkably similar.

USING LOGLINEAR ANALYSIS TO THE BEST ADVANTAGE

Loglinear analysis is not a panacea for all research problems with categorical data. Proper use of the method, as with any statistical method, requires thoughtful planning based on substantive knowledge and familiarity with the tool. Fienberg (1981, p. 58) discusses the various methods of the construction of hierarchical

Table 5

Effect Sizes In Predicting Outcome

For Selected Models

Models with Gender, Illness a

Effect		Outside	Self	Family
1. Gender X Outcome	Tau	2.3	2.2	2.2
	Beta	0.8	0.8	0.8
2. Illness X Outcome	Tau	3.5	3.3	3.5
	Beta	1.6	1.6	1.6
3. Outside X Outcome	Tau	1.7		
	Beta	1.2		
4. Self X Outcome	Tau		2.1	
	Beta		1.3	
5. Family X Outcome	Tau			2.1
	Beta			1.2

Coding Scheme for interpretation of effect sizes:

Gender (1=Male, 2=Female)
Outcome(1=Moderate Drinker, 2=Other)
Illness(1=Low, 2=High)
Labels (0=No, 1=Yes)

From Combs-Orme, Helzer, & Miller, 1987/88.

models. Some examples illustrate how loglinear analysis may be used in a less than ideal manner.

Richardson (1984) used data from a thematic apperception interview given to two large samples in 1957 and 1976 to look at attitudes toward friendship in women. It appears that two errors were made in the use of loglinear analysis in this study. First, the author ran a series of bivariate tests before using loglinear analysis to examine higher order effects. It is difficult to determine exactly how many tests were run, but it appears to be at least 15. Such tests are not only superfluous since loglinear analysis provides estimates of the bivariate relationships, but the use of multiple tests can seriously inflate the Type I error rate. A similar procedure was used by Zimmerman and Chein (1981), who ran 16 bivariate tests on data regarding various factors that influence decision-making in juvenile court cases before using loglinear analysis to test the fit of various models.

A more serious problem with the Richardson (1984) study, however, is that the testing of models appears, in contrast to the Brown (1983) study, to have been conducted without planning based on theoretical predictions or questions. The author presents no rationale for the numerous models that were tested, although such a rationale may have existed. The ability to test numerous models does not justify their being tested in the absence of a theoretical rationale.

Both the Richardson (1984) and the Zimmerman and Chein (1981) studies exhibit another undesirable feature. The failure of the authors in these studies to present estimates of the model parameters (that is, effect sizes for the significant variables in the model) prevents the reader from drawing conclusions about the relative strength of relationships among the variables. This is a serious omission because from a theoretical and practical point of view, most readers attach less importance to the adequacy of a model's fit than they do to the substantive interpretations of the effects of important factors in the model.

Computer Packages and References

Procedures are available for running loglinear analysis on all of the mainframe and personal computer statistical packages that are most commonly used by social work researchers (SPSS, SAS, and BMDP). The LOGLINEAR procedure in SPSS-X (Norusis, 1988) is particularly appealing because the manual is well written and includes not just information on running the program, but on the statistical method itself and interpretation of output. This is especially helpful to the reader who is not familiar with the notation. It should be noted that there are differences among the programs and among different texts in the type of notation used and the output that is produced. The reader should be familiar with the notation produced by his or her package and its comparability to any loglinear texts that are consulted.

There are a number of texts available to the reader who desires to be more familiar with the computational methods behind loglinear analysis. A standard guide that is simply written and widely used has been provided by Knoke and Burke (1980). Wickens's (1989) recent text also is easy to read, and includes more background and explanation. It is particularly helpful in relating loglinear analysis to other statistical methods and general statistical theory. Fienberg (1981) provides an informative history of analytical methods for cross-classified data, as well as particularly good examples.

Other references are more laborious to read and presume considerable statistical sophistication. Goodman's works (1971, 1972, 1979) provide an understanding of how the method was developed, but most readers will find them quite difficult. Bishop, Fienberg, and Holland's (1975) text is a classic, but it is also quite difficult. Agresti (1990) is also quite complex, but contains some particularly interesting examples. As loglinear analysis gains in popularity in the social sciences, new alternatives will no doubt emerge.

In summary, loglinear analysis is a statistical method for categorical independent and dependent variables. It has distinct advantages over both multiple contingency tests, which may fail to reveal complex interactions among the variables, and multiple regression, for which important assumptions may be violated. Although it does not solve all the problems one may have in conducting research with categorical data, loglinear analysis is a valuable and underused tool for social work researchers.

NOTES

1. Wickens (1989) provides an excellent discussion of three different conceptual meanings of unrelatedness, but all have the same practical outcomes for purposes of analysis with two-way tables.
2. The methodology of the Brown study suffers from the problem of violation of the assumption of independent observations, since the sample consisted of 33 couples whose opinions cannot be presumed to be independent, but the study is still an excellent example of partitioning.

REFERENCES

Agresti, A. (1990). *Categorical data analysis.* New York: John Wiley & Sons.
Aneshensel, C. S. (1983). An application of log-linear models: The stress-buffering function of alcohol use. *Journal of Drug Education, 13,* 287-301.
Bishop, Y., Fienberg, S. E., & Holland, P. W. (1975). *Discrete multivariate analysis: Theory and practice.* Cambridge, MA: The MIT Press.
Brown, S. V. (1983). The commitment and concerns of black adolescent parents. *Social Work Research and Abstracts, 19*(4), 27-34.
Cleary, P. D. & Angel, R. (1984). The analysis of relationships involving dichotomous dependent variables. *Journal of Health and Social Behavior, 25,* 334-348.
Cohen, J. & Cohen, P. (1983). *Applied multiple regression/Correlation analysis for the behavioral sciences.* 2nd ed. Hillsdale, NJ: Lawrence Erlbaum Associates, Publishers.
Combs-Orme, T., Helzer, J. E., & Miller, R. H. (1987/88). The application of labeling theory to alcoholism. *Journal of Social Service Research, 11,* 73-91.
Fienberg, S. E. (1981). *The analysis of cross-classified data.* 2nd ed. Cambridge, MA: The MIT Press.
Fleiss, J. L. (1981). *Statistical methods for rates and proportions.* New York: John Wiley & Sons.

Fleiss, J. L., Williams, J. B. W., & Dubro, A. F. (1986). The logistic regression analysis of psychiatric data. *Journal of Psychiatric Research, 20,* 145-209.

Goodman, L. A. (1971). The analysis of multidimensional contingency tables: Stepwise procedures and direct estimation methods for building models for multiple classifications. *Technometrics, 13,* 33-61.

Goodman, L. A. (1972). A general model for the analysis of surveys. *American Journal of Sociology, 77,* 1035-1086.

Goodman, L. A. (1979). A brief guide to the causal analysis of data from surveys. *American Journal of Sociology, 84,* 1078-1095.

Hays, W. L. (1988). *Statistics.* 4th ed. New York: Holt, Rinehart and Winston, Inc.

Hughes, S., Johnson, K., Rosenbaum, S., Simons, J., & Butler, E. (1987). *The health of America's children: Maternal and child health data book.* Washington, D. C.: Children's Defense Fund.

Jenkins, S., Diamond, B. E., Flanzraich, M., Gibson, J. W., Hendricks, J., & Marshood, N. (1983). Ethnic differentials in foster care placements. *Social Work Research and Abstracts* (4), *19,* 41-45.

Knoke, D. & Burke, P. (1980). *Log-linear models.* Beverly Hills: Sage Publications.

Norusis, M. J. (1988). *SPSS-X advanced statistics guide.* Chicago: SPSS, Inc.

Richardson, V. (1984). Clinical-historical aspects of friendship deprivation among women. *Social Work Research and Abstracts, 20*(1), 19-24.

Rosenberg, M. (1968). *The logic of survey analysis.* New York: Basic Books, Inc.

Wickens, T. D. (1989). *Multiway contingency tables analysis for the social sciences.* Hillsdale, New Jersey: Lawrence Erlbaum Associates, Publishers.

Zimmerman, M. K. & Chein, D. B. (1981). Decision making in the juvenile court. *Social Work Research and Abstracts, 17*(4), 14-21.

Event History Analysis: A Proportional Hazards Perspective on Modeling Outcomes in Intensive Family Preservation Services

Mark W. Fraser
Peter J. Pecora
Chirapat Popuang
David A. Haapala

SUMMARY. This paper demonstrates the use of event history analysis and reports on the correlates of service outcomes for the HOMEBUILDERS model of Intensive Family Preservation Services (IFPS). The paper focuses on the use of the proportional hazards model, the assumption of proportionality, methods for dealing with violations of proportionality, and implications for collecting event data.

This paper has two purposes: (1) to demonstrate the application of a relatively new statistical procedure called event history analysis (also survival analysis,

Mark W. Fraser holds a PhD in Social Welfare from the University of Washington, Seattle, WA. He is Associate professor at the Graduate School of Social Work, University of Utah, where he directs the School's PhD Program. His recent work has focused on family preservation services and research education in social work. With David Haapala and Peter Pecora, he is a co-author of *Families in Crisis: The Impact of Intensive Family Preservation Services* (Fraser, M.W., Pecora, P.J., & Haapala, D.A.) (1991). Hawthorne, NY: Aldine de Gruyter. The results of his research in child welfare, delinquency prevention, and substance abuse have been published in many different journals.

Peter J. Pecora holds a PhD in Social Welfare from the University of Washington in Seattle. He is the Manager of Research with The Casey Family Program, and Associate Professor at the School of Social Work, University of Washington. The co-author of three books on personnel management and program evaluation in child welfare, as well as the recent book, *Families in Crisis: The Impact of Intensive Family Preservation Services* (Fraser, M.W., Pecora, P.J., & Haapala, D.A.) (1991) Hawthorne, NY: Aldine de Gruyter, the results of his research have been published in a variety of professional journals.

© 1992 by The Haworth Press, Inc. All rights reserved.

Cox regression, and failure-time analysis); and (2) to describe risk factors for placement in a sample of families that received treatment from the HOMEBUILDERS™ Intensive Family Preservation Services (IFPS) program. Based on clinical and program data from a prospective study of 409 children from 312 families that received IFPS, the correlates of treatment success/failure are estimated using event history analysis (EHA). While event history analysis will be discussed in general, the assumptions and procedures common to the Proportional Hazards (PH) Model of EHA are the focus of this paper. In the course of demonstrating the use of the PH model, findings that extend our previous work on the risk factors for IFPS treatment are presented.

THE USE OF EVENTS AS SERVICE OUTCOMES

In the sense that an outcome is regressed on a linear combination of explanatory variables, EHA is usually described as regression-like analysis for longitudinal data. Suggesting its potential, the outcomes used in EHA may be almost any kind of discrete event for which information is routinely collected. In many agencies, for example, it is typical to classify clients as "service failures"

Chirapat Popuang holds a Masters Degree in Sociology from the University of Utah, where he is a doctoral candidate. Mr. Popuang has conducted research in the areas of family preservation services, refugee resettlement, and fertility.

David A. Haapala holds a PhD in Psychology from the Saybrook Institute. He is the co-founder and Executive Director of Behavioral Sciences Institute, a nonprofit corporation to provide, promote, and study community-based family-centered services. He is the author of numerous papers on program evaluation, social service delivery, and public policy in child welfare. He is a co-author of two recent books: *Keeping Families Together: The Homebuilders Model* (Kinney, J., Haapala, D.A., & Booth, C.) (1991). Hawthorne, NY: Aldine de Gruyter; and *Families in Crisis: The Impact of Intensive Family Preservation Services* (Fraser, M.W., Pecora, P.J., & Haapala, D.A.) (1991). Hawthorne, NY: Aldine de Gruyter.

This paper is adapted, in part, from "Assessing the Risks of Treatment Failure in Intensive Family Preservation Services," a paper presented by Mark Fraser, Katherine McDade, David Haapala, and Peter Pecora for the Second Annual Research Conference, Children's Mental Health Services and Policy: Building a Research Base, Tampa, FL (February 27, 1989). The research on which this paper is based was made possible through grants from the Office of Human Development Services, Administration for Children, Youth, and Families, U. S. Department of Health and Human Services (No. 90-CW-0731) and the Edna McConnell Clark Foundation.

Requests for reprints should be sent to Mark W. Fraser, Graduate School of Social Work, University of Utah, Salt Lake City, UT 84112.

because of the occurrence of a critical life event such as a hospitalization, an arrest, a relapse, a victimization, or death. Conversely, the absence of an event is often the basis for declaring service to be successful (for examples, see Bienen & Van De Walle, 1989; Slonim-Nevo & Clark, 1989). In most IFPS research, the placement of a child in substitute care (foster care, group home, residential treatment, etc.) is used to classify family treatment as successful (in the absence of placement) or unsuccessful (in the presence of placement). Then discriminant analysis is used to identify factors that distinguish children who were placed from those who were not (Nelson, 1990; Nelson & Associates, 1988; Yuan & Associates, 1990).

This approach has serious limitations. The standard deviations in success and failure groups may be different, creating heteroscedasticity and confounding the estimation of statistical significance. As important, however, the use of binary outcome measures–the occurrence or absence of a critical event such as placement out of the home–sacrifices a substantial amount of information regarding the length of time that children in "failure" families may have been living successfully and safely in their homes.

Further, information may be sacrificed or lost because some children and their families fail to complete a follow-up period; they move or simply decline to participate in long-term follow-ups and are "lost" to studies. Often these clients are called "dropouts" and are excluded from analyses, examined only for bias due to mortality. By using an event history approach, partial data from such subjects may be included in analyses. Because of this and because EHA breaks away from reliance on periodic dates of data collection (as in traditional panel studies)–that is, it makes use of information on the length of time that clients "survive" until the *exact* date of a failure event–event history analysis has become a powerful quantitative method for the analysis of case file, MIS, and other longitudinal data (Campbell, Mutran, & Parker, 1986).

Survival or Event History Analysis

In the analysis of event data, time is a critical variable. Survival to the occurrence of an event such as a placement may be measured in hours, days, or weeks. Expressed as the rate at which events occur within a time period, time and events are conjoined as the dependent measure in EHA. For example, evaluators of a Child Protective Services Treatment Project might measure abuse events subsequent to treatment. By collecting official and self-reported data on abuse events, a probability of abuse for each day of survival after the termination of treatment might be estimated. Discussed in subsequent sections of this paper, a transformation of this survival rate would become the dependent measure in event history analysis.

There are numerous EHA models and evaluators must choose one. Each model is based on different survival and density functions with different assumptions regarding the shape of the survival distribution. These include an exponential distribution where one assumes that the risk of an event over time is invariant, as well as the Weibull, log-logistic, gamma, and Gompertz distributions where the risk of an event is assumed to change over time. Different distributions represent different survival patterns.

The choice of a distribution or model is based on the shape of the survival function across time. Survivor functions express the probability that an individual survives until time t, that is that placement or some other event has not yet occurred at some point in time. Survivor functions do not increase over time and will gradually approach zero. But they can take different shapes. As indicated in Figure 1a, for example, human beings have a survival function that shows relatively lower mortality in the mid years of life, with higher mortality that gradually approaches 100% in later years.

As indicated in Figures 1b through 1d, there are a variety of alternative survival patterns (Blossfeld, Hamerle, & Mayer, 1989, pp. 26-42), and one tries to select an EHA model by matching the shape of a known survival pattern to the expected distribution of survival in a population of interest. To use the exponential model, for example, one would plot the probability of survival by time and expect to observe a function similar to that shown in Figure 1b. The Weibull, log-logistic, and other distributions are somewhat more flexible. They have shape parameters (alpha) that may be altered for different survival patterns. Notice how the survival curves become steeper as the value of alpha increases for the Weibull distribution (Figure 1c) and log-logistic distribution (Figure 1d) (Kalbfleisch & Prentice, 1980, pp. 21-30). Weibull and log-logistic survival functions with higher alphas might be used to model the rapid mortality observed in some diseases, the high failure rate of poorly engineered automobiles, or the high recidivism rates of some early release correctional programs.

Transforming the Survival Function to a Hazard Rate

Across time, the odds for a placement (or any other event) may be transformed into a "hazard" function given by:

$$h(t) = \lim_{s \to 0} P(t, t+s)/s \qquad [1]$$

or the probability that an individual experiences an event in the time interval t to $(t + s)$, given that an individual was at risk at time t, and where s is an interval length greater than 0. As s becomes smaller and approaches zero, the ratio reaches a limit. In the case of IFPS research, the hazard function [1] represents the time-to-failure for each child in the study because it is based on the odds of placement for each child for each day of participation in treatment and the follow-up period, or alternatively, for each day of risk of placement.

Like survival functions, hazard functions have different shapes that should be used to select an event history model which fits a set of observed data. Shown in Figure 2, the observed hazard rate for human mortality reflects the higher probabilities of death faced by infants and the aging.

FIGURE 1

Survival Function for Human Mortality, Exponential Distribution,
Weibull Distribution, and Log-Logistic Distribution

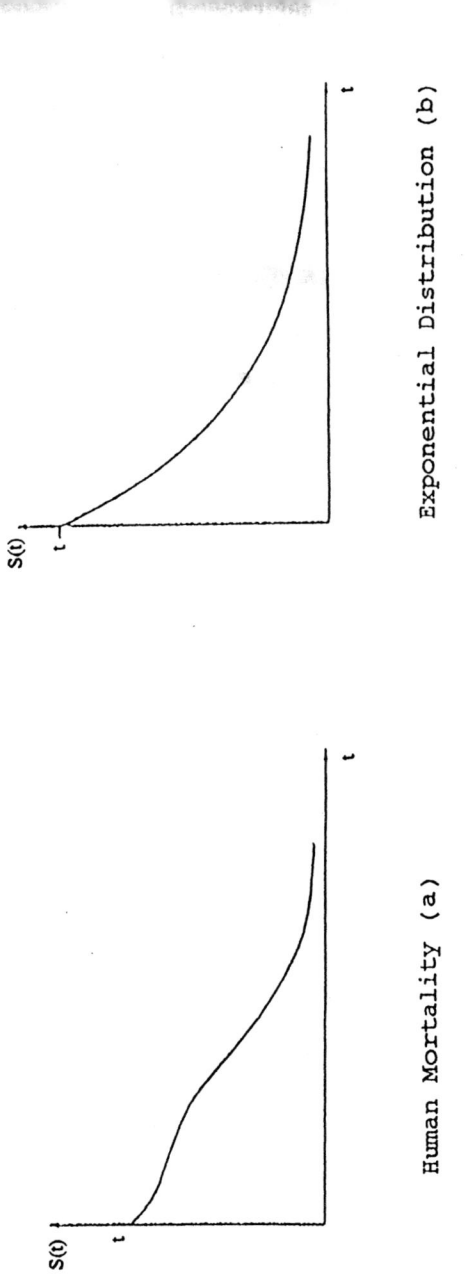

Human Mortality (a)

Exponential Distribution (b)

FIGURE 1 (continued)

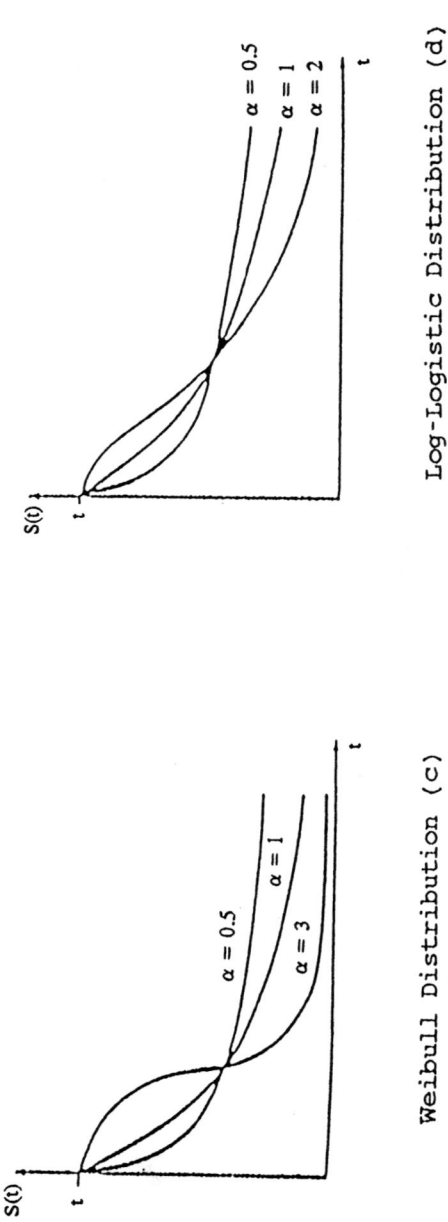

Weibull Distribution (c)

Log-Logistic Distribution (d)

Source: Blossfeld, H. P., Hamerle, A., Mayer, K. U. (1989). *Event history analysis: Statistical theory and application in the social sciences.* Hillsdale, NJ: Lawrence Erlbaum Associates, Publishers, pp. 32-41.

The hazard rates for the exponential, Weibull, and log-logistic models are also shown in Figure 2. Notice that the exponential model is equivalent to the Weibull model with alpha set to 1. To select a model, say, for human mortality, one would examine the human mortality hazard rate and compare it with the hazard rates in Figures 1b to 1d. As is often the case, there appears to be no particularly good fit.

Hazard Models

Each hazard may be expressed algebraically as a model (Allison, 1984, pp. 22-25). The hazard rate for the exponential distribution shows the constant or invariant risk model:

$$\ln h(t) = a + b_1 x_{1i} + \ldots + b_p x_{pi} \qquad [2]$$

where $x_{1i}, \ldots, x_{pi}$ = the explanatory variables of the ith case in the sample; and
where $b_1, b_2, \ldots, b_p$ = regression coefficients for variables 1 to p (the last explanatory variable).

Because time is not included as an explanatory variable in the exponential model (risk is assumed to be the same over time), it may be unacceptable for many applications. We know, for example, that the hazard for human mortality varies over time and thus the exponential distribution would be a poor choice if one wanted to model mortality. Similarly, we might expect that the risk of placement would accelerate steeply after the termination of IFPS services and, consequently, the exponential model would not provide a good fit for IFPS data.

Other models offer greater flexibility. Shown in Figures 2c and 2d, the Weibull and log-logistic hazard rates may be used to model probabilities that vary over time. The Weibull model, for example, may be expressed as:

$$\ln h(t) = a + b_1 x_{1i} + \ldots + b_p x_{pi} + c \ln(t) \qquad [3]$$

where c must be less than -1 and $\ln(t)$ is the natural log of time. There are many other models and our aim here is only to exemplify the process of selecting an EHA approach. As with survival functions, hazard rate alphas indicate alternative shape parameters. By setting the Weibull alpha parameter at a value of 3, for example, one might model steeply accelerating placements subsequent to the termination of services. This model might provide a good fit for IFPS data, if we were to observe little success in preventing out-of-home placements. Alternatively, a decreasing monotone is produced by setting alpha to values less than 1 (and, conversely, an increasing monotone is produced by setting alpha at values greater than 1) (Blossfeld, Hamerle, & Mayer, 1989, pp. 26-42; Kalbfleisch & Prentice, 1980, pp. 21-30). As indicated in Figure 2d, alphas from the log-logistic distribution may be used to model still different hazard rates.

FIGURE 2

Hazard Function for Human Mortality, Exponential Distribution,
Weibull Distribution, and Log-Logistic Distribution

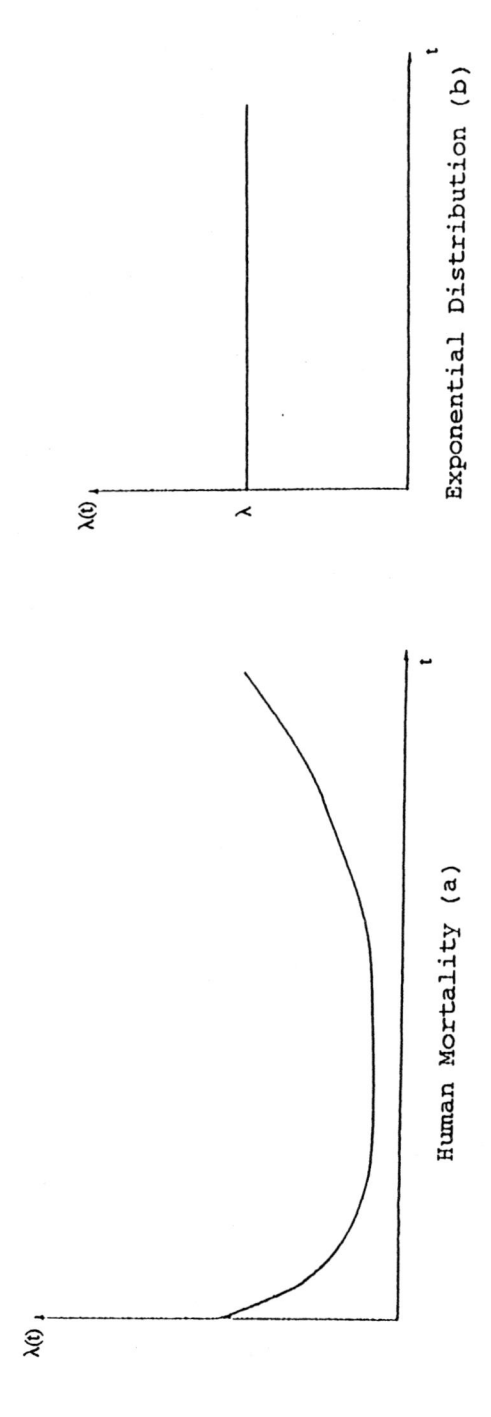

Human Mortality (a)

Exponential Distribution (b)

Weibull Distribution (c)

Log-Logistic Distribution (d)

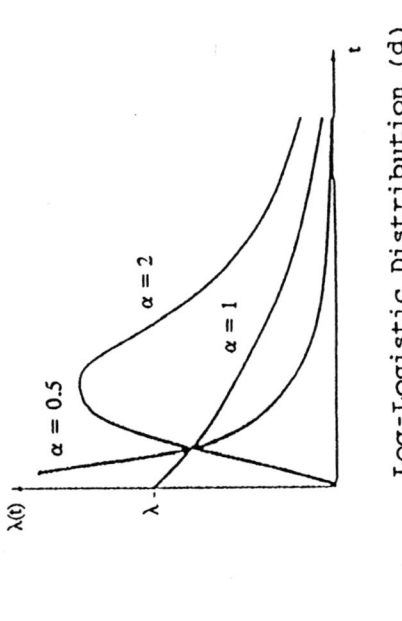

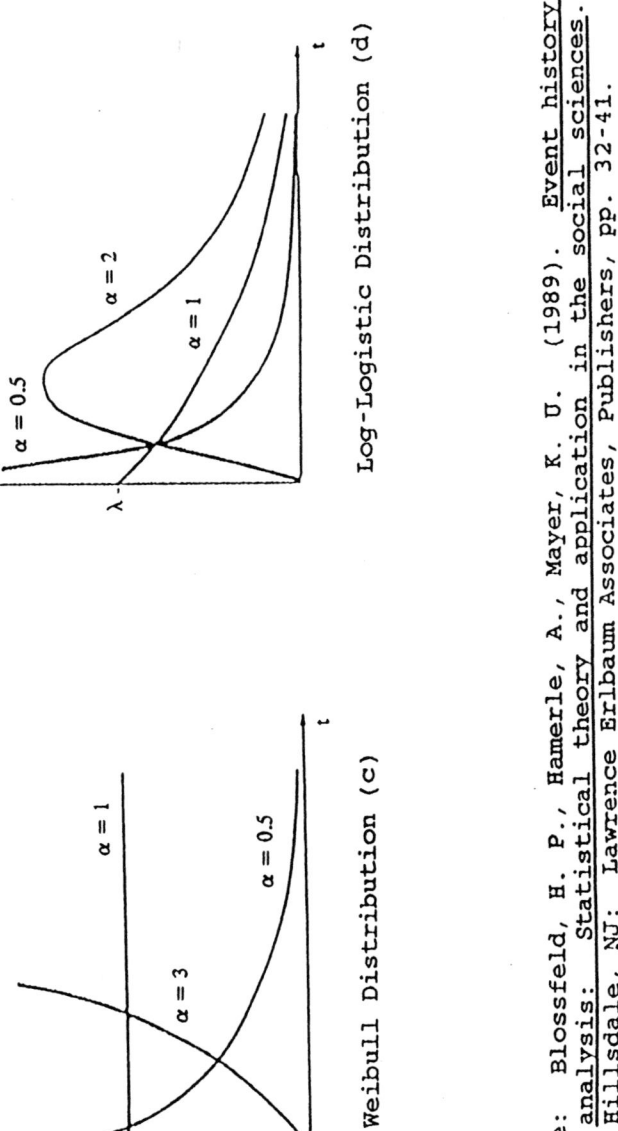

Source: Blossfeld, H. P., Hamerle, A., Mayer, K. U. (1989). Event history analysis: Statistical theory and application in the social sciences. Hillsdale, NJ: Lawrence Erlbaum Associates, Publishers, pp. 32-41.

The Proportional Hazards Model

In this paper, the Cox event history analysis model called the Proportional Hazards procedure will be demonstrated. It has an important advantage: it requires no assumptions about the overall shape of the survival or hazard function. However, it also has an important limitation: it requires that the risk of placement remain constant for all individuals at risk. This is called the "proportionality" assumption and we will examine it in this paper. With covariates, the PH model takes the form of:

$$\ln h(t) = a(t) + b_1 x_{1i} + \ldots + b_p x_{pi} \quad [4]$$

where $a(t)$ is any function of time, so long as the ratio of hazards is constant for any two individuals at any point in time (the proportionality assumption).

In many texts, the PH model is expressed as (Hopkins, 1988, p. 719):

$$h(t;z) = h_0(t) \, EXP(b'z) \quad [5]$$

where b = a vector of unknown regression coefficients;
z = a vector of "covariates" or explanatory variables; and
$h_0(t)$ = an unknown hazard function for an individual with covariate vector z = 0.

The PH model makes the assumption that the relationship between the hazard rate and the log-linear function of explanatory variables is multiplicative. This implies that the ratio of hazard functions for two individuals will not change over time, that it is not dependent on time. That is,

$$\ln [\, h(t;z) / h_0(t) \,] = b'z \quad [6]$$

If so, then one concludes that the Proportionality Assumption is satisfied.

Partial Likelihood Estimation

Common to all event history models, the hazard is used computationally as an outcome measure. In the PH model, regression coefficients for variables that explain or alter the hazard are estimated using a procedure called "partial likelihood estimation." Partial likelihood is based on the division of the likelihood function into two factors (Allison, 1984, pp. 67-71). The first factor depends on the order in which events occur. It contains information about the covariates. The second factor depends on the exact times that events occur. In 1972, Cox developed a procedure that involved discarding the second factor and using the first factor as the basis for the estimation of regression coefficients (Cox, 1972, 1975). He and others have been able to show that the loss of efficiency due to the use of event order rather than precise time is minimal, so long as the ratio of hazards is time invariant for any two individuals. This is the basis for the proportionality assumption and the term "Proportional Hazards Model." The approach has nonparametric properties because of its reliance on event order and is occasionally referred to as "semi-parametric." It produces asymptotically unbiased and normally distributed regression estimates (Lawless, 1982).

Time-Varying Explanatory Variables

Each EHA model-including the PH model-can be generalized to allow the failure rate to be a function of explanatory variables that vary over time. The use of time-varying explanatory variables distinguishes EHA from many other regression-like procedures. Covariates that vary over time are often theoretically relevant. In IFPS research, for example, school attendance by week might be used as a covariate under the hypothesis that truancy is correlated with the likelihood of placement. Readers are cautioned, however, that the inclusion of time-varying covariates greatly increases the complexity of the estimation procedure.

Unobserved Heterogeneity

Most EHA models do not contain an error term and unobserved heterogeneity may influence the hazard rate. This is an important limitation of the EHA approach, for EHA models assume that the covariates fully explain the hazard. Where a particular distribution is assumed (as in exponential, Weibull, and log-logistic models) and even where it is not (as in the PH model), findings may be spurious when important variables have been omitted from the model. For example, suppose that after school employment affects placement rates in the sense that the hazards for children who are and are not employed after school are quite different. If after school employment is unmeasured and omitted from the model, the estimated hazard may poorly approximate the true hazard for placement.

On balance, unobserved heterogeneity appears to produce a declining hazard rate. Thus, when the hazard declines, caution is warranted (Allison, 1988; Blossfeld, Hamerle, & Mayer, 1989). Much of the current research on EHA is focusing on the development of parameter estimation procedures that contain error terms and the development of tests for unobserved heterogeneity (Blossfeld, Hamerle, & Mayer, 1989, pp. 91-104). This work involves procedures to estimate and test residuals in a fashion that is similar to residuals analysis in ordinary least squares (OLS) regression (Blossfeld & Hamerle, 1988; Blossfeld, Hamerle, & Mayer, 1989). At present, readers are cautioned to develop models that have construct validity and to condition EHA-based conclusions on the developmental stage of the EHA technology.

HOMEBUILDERS: Brief and Intensive Home-Based Family Treatment

As suggested initially, event history analysis is used in this paper to identify factors associated with the placement of children whose families participated in the HOMEBUILDERS model of IFPS. Critics and advocates have recently renewed their long-standing challenge to child welfare agencies to develop innovative services to strengthen families, keeping them together, while protecting children and preventing unnecessary out-of-home placements (Edna McConnell Clark Foundation, 1985, p. 2; Rzepnicki, 1987). Intensive Family Preservation Services are one response to this challenge (Whittaker, Kinney, Tracy, & Booth, 1990). They represent a refinement and extension of family-based treatment provided in the 1950s to "multi-problem" families (Geismar & Ayers, 1958; Horejsi, 1981). They are designed to stabilize crises, protect children, strengthen family ties, build parents' child management skills, and augment families' tangible resources (AuClaire & Schwartz, 1986; Callister, Mitchell, & Tolley, 1986; Compher, 1983; Jones, Newman, & Shyne, 1976; Kinney, Haapala, Booth, & Leavitt, 1990). IFPS are not a "cure" for child abuse or other serious child- and parent-related problems, and they cannot replace the need for out-of-home care for children (Magura, 1981; Stein, 1985). But in the continuum of services for families and children, IFPS are increasingly viewed as a practical alternative to placement (Frankel, 1988; Hinckley & Ellis, 1985; Jones, 1985; Whittaker et al., 1990).

The HOMEBUILDERS program is distinguished from other family preservation services by its intensity and diversity (Haapala & Kinney, 1988; Kinney, Haapala, Booth, & Leavitt, in press). HOMEBUILDERS therapists provide a wide range of counseling, advocacy, training, and concrete assistance to families. They work with families in the home and services are directed toward placement prevention.

Small caseloads and brief, intensive services. HOMEBUILDERS therapists carry small caseloads of two families at a time, and they provide 24 hours-a-day case coverage. Treatment for families accepted by HOMEBUILDERS begins within a day of referral. Services are crisis oriented, intensive and brief. On average, they are provided for only four weeks, and it is not uncommon for the workers to spend 10 hours a week with a family.

Skills training and concrete assistance. The HOMEBUILDERS program is based upon cognitive-behavioral, crisis, ecological, and Rogerian theories. The family and its social support system are viewed as the focus of service. Workers place an emphasis upon solving problems identified by family members. They view themselves as supportive, teaching "colleagues" of family members. Training and teaching focuses on child management, bargaining, contracting, active listening, modeling, values clarification, and problem-solving (Kinney, Haapala, Booth, & Leavitt, 1990, in press; Kinney, Madsen, Flemming, & Haapala, 1977). HOMEBUILDERS therapists also provide or arrange for a variety of concrete services to assist families to obtain food, clothing, housing, medicine, employment, day care, and transportation. Although the evidence is not conclusive (Yuan & Associates, 1990) and more experimental work is needed, studies suggest that HOME-BUILDERS and IFPS programs similar to HOMEBUILDERS are effective in preventing placements (Fixsen, Olivier, & Blase, 1990; Fraser, Pecora, & Haapala, in press; Haapala & Kinney, 1988; Hinckley & Ellis, 1985).

Outcome Measures in IFPS Programs

A variety of outcome criteria have been used in examining the effectiveness of IFPS and other family-based services. Measures proximal to the family often focus on child behaviors such as school attendance, delinquent behavior, and household rule compliance. Other outcome measures focus on parenting skills, home conditions, and family dynamics, while still others focus on conditions related to family functioning such as parental employment and social support.

Although such proximal outcome measures are important, the prevention of unnecessary placements has received the greatest amount of attention by evaluators. Placement prevention has been, and continues to be, an important, policy-relevant goal of IFPS. Yet in spite of its predominance, many issues remain to be resolved regarding the use of placement as an outcome measure:

> Of the many negative service outcomes that are possible for children, which living situations (foster care, group care, psychiatric hospital, runaway, living with friends, etc.) should be defined as placements?

> What criteria should be used to distinguish "necessary" from "unnecessary" placements?

> What is a reasonable length of time to expect a brief, crisis oriented service to affect the lives of service recipients?

The lack of common definitions of placement and consistent follow-up periods seriously compromises the literature on family preservation programs. Notwithstanding, placement prevention remains an outcome of unique importance because of the presumed lower costs associated with serving children successfully.

METHOD

Research Participants

To identify risk factors for service failure and to demonstrate the utility of the PH approach, case information from a prospective study of child welfare clients is used. Data were collected at HOMEBUILDERS intake and case closure from 312 families, including 409 children who constitute the unit of analysis. A total of four HOMEBUILDERS program sites were used in the State of Washington (Snohomish, Pierce, King, and Spokane counties). These program sites served a variety of urban, suburban, and rural clients, with the Spokane and Pierce sites serving more rural families.

Family functioning and child placement information was collected 12 months after IFPS intake from 187 families (including 245 children) that had entered treatment sufficiently early in the course of the study to be eligible for inclusion in a one-year follow-up. The remaining 125 families (with 164 children) were tracked until the follow-up period ended in August, 1987. The follow-up times for children from these 125 families varied from 1 to 11 months; no child was tracked for the full 12-month period. In traditional data analysis, one would classify all 164 children from these families as "drop-outs" or cases with incomplete data. They would be eliminated from the data set; however, using EHA we are able to include them in the analysis.

Placement Events as the Dependent Variable

Because IFPS are designed to strengthen families and prevent child placements, a service failure event was defined to include any child placement in substitute care–such as a foster or group home–or any out-of-home episode–such as running away or leaving home to live with friends–of two weeks, duration or more. The absence of an out-of-home episode by this criterion was defined as service success. For each child, time-to-placement in days was recorded, if a placement occurred.

Child placement episodes were monitored through computerized information systems that tracked placement payments by public agencies. In addition, placements were identified by maintaining contacts with referring and IFPS workers, and by conducting interviews with primary caretakers at service termination and at the end of the twelve month follow-up period.

Intake Criteria and Referring Agencies

Families were eligible for service if, and only if, one or more of their children was deemed at "risk of imminent placement." To meet this criterion, referring agencies must have been planning to place a child within one week. Workers from Children's Protective Services (CPS) (serving children in danger of abuse or neglect) and Family Reconciliation Services (serving ungovernable children and families in conflict) from the Washington State Department of Social and Health Services referred families to HOMEBUILDERS. According to public policy, referrals could be made only when children were in danger of imminent out-of-home placement. CPS referrals accounted for 45.5% of all referrals and the remainder came from Family Reconciliation Services.

Eligibility for IFPS was contingent also upon reasonable assurances that a child's safety could be ensured, and that at least one parent was willing to schedule an initial appointment with the HOMEBUILDERS worker. All referrals were screened for appropriateness on the basis of these criteria by a HOMEBUILDERS intake coordinator.

Explanatory Variables:
Measures of Child, Parent, and Family Functioning

Family characteristics. Based on self-reports from parents, IFPS therapists, and children, family functioning and case outcomes were assessed a variety of different ways. Items from the Child Welfare League of America's Family Risk Scales (FRS) were used to measure changes in various aspects of child, parent, and family functioning (Magura & Moses, 1986). Each response category for each item is fully anchored by two to five sentence descriptions. Items focus on parenting capacity, individual (both parent and child) functioning, and environmental conditions that have shown to be associated with out-of-home placement and are potentially altered through treatment (Magura, Moses, & Jones, 1987).

Social and demographic data. Demographic data were collected by treatment and intake workers for all families participating in the study. These data included: (a) primary and secondary (if one) child caretaker age, gender, and years of education; (b) ethnicity/race; (c) family structure; (d) source of referral; (e) religious affiliation and involvement; (f) source and amount of income; (g) ages of children; (h) number of prior placements (if any); (i) school attendance at the time of intake; (j) drug/alcohol use of children at intake; and other information. These data are selectively presented in Table 1 (for a full description, please see Fraser, Pecora, & Haapala, in press).

Treatment goal achievement. In addition, data were collected on case and service characteristics including the type and amount of clinical and concrete services provided, treatment goals, and the amount of in-person and telephone contact with clients. In conjunction with the IFPS therapists and supervisors, a checklist of commonly used treatment goals was developed. The Goal Checklist contained 16 parent- and child-related behaviorally-anchored goals. Goals for parents focused on increasing parenting, anger management, conflict resolution, and communication skills as well as improving household conditions, developing greater trust within the family, and decreasing depression, anxiety, and fear. For children goals focused on decreasing delinquent behavior, running away, and alcohol/drug use, as well as increasing compliance with household rules and improving school attendance or performance. At the start of treatment, workers checked-off all the goals that were part of each family's case plan, and at the close of treatment, they rated the achievement of each goal using a five-point scale of: (1) no progress, (2) about 25% achieved, (3) about half achieved, (4) about 75% achieved, and (5) totally achieved. Across all goals specified for each family, an index of "mean goal achievement" was computed.

Table 1
Parent (Caretaker), Family, and Child Characteristics:
Measures of Central Tendency*

PARENT CHARACTERISTICS

Primary Caretaker (n=311)
Age (Years)	($\underline{M}$)	35.0
	(SD)	(6.7)
Female (%)		93.2%
Education (Years)	$\underline{M}$	12.4
	(SD)	(2.1)

Secondary Caretaker (n=155)
Age (Years)	$\underline{M}$	37.5
	(SD)	(10.0)
Female (%)		3.5%
Education (Years)	$\underline{M}$	13.0
	(SD)	(2.3)

FAMILY CHARACTERISTICS

Household Size	$\underline{M}$	4.3
	(SD)	(1.6)
Number of children at home	$\underline{M}$	2.6
	(SD)	(1.2)

Asian, Black, Hispanic,
and other Minorities Served (%) 18.3%

Family Structure (%)
- Birthparents together 17.7%
- Single parent, divorce or separation 36.7%
- Birthparent with stepparent 19.3%
- Birthparent living with other adult 12.5%
- Single, never married 5.8%
- Other 8.0%

Case Referral Source (%)
- Child Protective Services 45.5%
- Family Reconciliation Services 54.5%

Mean Number of Address Changes
in Last Five Years (SD) 2.4
 (2.3)

Renting Home (%) 61.2%

PARENT CHARACTERISTICS

Caretaker Living Arrangements (%)
    Living together, married   39.9%
    Living together, unmarried   11.6%
    Not living together   11.6%
    Single caretaker   35.7%
    Other   1.3%

Family Gross Income (%)
    $5,000 and under   10.1%
    5,001 - 10,000   33.2%
    10,001 - 15,000   16.9%
    15,001 - 20,000   15.0%
    20,001 - 25,000   6.8%
    25,001 - 30,000   6.5%
    Over 30,000   11.4%

Major Source of Family Income (%)
    Job   62.8%
    Social Security   3.2%
    Income Assistance (e.g., GA, AFDC)   29.1%
    Retirement   .0%
    Unemployment   1.3%
    None   .3%
    Other   3.2%

CHILD CHARACTERISTICS

Age of children at risk

Oldest Child (n=233)	M		11.9
	(SD)		(4.3)
Second oldest (n=129)	M		9.5
	(SD)		(4.9)
Third oldest (n=47)	M		7.7
	(SD)		(4.5)

Prior placements of children at risk

Oldest child	M	.43
	(SD)	(0.8)
Second oldest	M	.38
	(SD)	(0.9)
Third oldest	M	.33
	(SD)	(0.7)

Months of prior placements (if one)

Oldest child	M	4.9
	(SD)	(6.7)
Second oldest	M	4.9
	(SD)	(5.8)
Third oldest	M	4.2
	(SD)	(4.0)

TABLE 1 (continued)

SELECTED FAMILY RISK FACTORS (dummy variables)

Proportion of parents with functioning impaired by mental illness; capacity to fulfill child caretaking role is limited	.158 (.24)
Proportion of parents who preferred out-of-home placement at intake; may have requested immediate child placement; willing to delay placement	.129 (.34)
Proportion of parents who seemed concerned but careless or indifferent about problems, rejected parental role at intake	.259 (.44)
Proportion of parents who seemed concerned but careless or indifferent about problems, rejected parental role at exit	.148 (.36)
Proportion where at least one family member is employed	.575 (.49)
Proportion of children whose physical needs are met marginally or inadequately at intake	.247 (.43)
Proportion of children whose physical needs are met marginally or inadequately at exit	.225 (.42)
Proportion of children in the home at intake	.905 (.29)
Proportion of children in the home at referral	.849 (.36)
Proportion of children age 13 to 17	.490 (.50)
Proportion of children who are ethnic or racial minority	.184 (.39)
Proportion of children with at least one prior out-of-home placement	.276 (.45)
Proportion of children with drug or alcohol involvement at intake	.237 (.43)
Proportion of children truant 50% or more	.251 (.43)
Proportion where parent rarely demonstrates affection and may reject child openly at intake	.240 (.43)

TREATMENT GOAL ACHIEVEMENT

Mean Treatment Goal Achievement (5 levels of goal achievement)	3.305 (.72)
Proportion with Modest (level 2 or greater) Mean Treatment Goal Achievement	.937 (.24)

SOCIAL SUPPORT (PRIMARY CARETAKER)

Coaching from extended family or other (at least twice a week)	.220 (.41)

*The n of cases varies slightly because of missing information.

Scaling Ordinal Variables

To promote the interpretation of the ordinal measures used in the FRS, many items were dichotomized by examining frequency distributions and service failure rates. This eliminated knotty problems interpreting changes in the hazard rate for unit changes in explanatory measures that were not interval in nature. By definition, unit changes in ordinal measures are not equal, and to make maximum use of regression procedures, it is desirable to use covariates at the interval level.

To create more readily interpretable findings, dichotomies were created. Binary FRS variables were created that maximized the odds of service failure across each variable, while preserving an adequate number of children in each category of the explanatory variables. For example, the ordinal FRS variable Physical Needs of Child had four response categories (each with its own unshown 2-4 sentence anchor statement): (1) physical needs adequately met; (2) physical needs marginally or inconsistently met, but little or no effect on child's functioning; (3) physical needs not being met, affecting child's functioning, but no illness; and (4) physical needs not met, serious illness or injury involved. By cutting the scale to create a dummy variable such that 1 = 0 and 2 to 4 = 1, the measure was "cornered" to produce the largest possible EHA t-ratio, while preserving an adequate number of cases in each of the two categories (Blossfeld, Hamerle, & Mayer, 1989, pp. 47-50).

Although family circumstances such as those described by the fourth category are likely to produce immediate out-of-home placement, the definition of a cornered variable must be conditioned on the distribution of children across all response categories. Because there were only six children who were rated as "4" in the sample, a score of "1" on the cornered variable might be interpreted as modest physical needs that warrant immediate intervention but not out-of-home placement. This measure is used in this report. To promote interpretability, other ordinal measures and some demographic measures with skewed distributions were scaled in a similar fashion.

Scaling Nonlinearities and Interpreting EHA Coefficients

PH model coefficients may be interpreted in the same way that OLS coefficients are interpreted (Blossfeld, Hamerle, & Mayer, 1989). That is, if the coefficient of an interval- or ratio-level variable such as AGE were to be positive, then one could argue that as age increases, the odds or risk of service failure increases. The exponentiated value of the coefficient is equivalent to the relative risk or change in the log-odds of placement for a unit change in an explanatory variable.

However, the odds of placement for some variables do not increase linearly. In this report, for example, we dichotomized AGE because the bivariate risk of placement by years of age increased significantly for teens, while it was about the same for children 12 years of age and less. When the risk of placement does not increase linearly with each change in value of a variable, it is appropriate to seek a better fit by using transformed variables, and one of the simplest, yet most policy-relevant transformations with regard to AGE, involves distinguishing teenagers from younger children. Since the etiology of adolescent behavior is usually more complex than the etiology of the behavior of younger children (in the sense that school and peer variables are often involved), AGE was dichotomized such that teens received a score of "1" and younger children received a score of "0." This transformation produced the highest odds of service failure by AGE (as indicated by the relative EHA t-values for various age groupings), suggesting that optimal value was achieved by creating a "teenager" dummy variable from the age data.

Assuming the coefficient for AGE was 2.0, one could say that children over the age of 12 are twice as likely to be placed as children 12 or less years of age. To estimate the relative risk as a percentage, the value 1.0 is subtracted from the exponentiated coefficient and the remainder is multiplied by 100. In such a case, it is possible to argue that the risk of placement is 100 percent greater, or twice as great, for adolescents.

Because the EHA model is multiplicative, the risk for multi-level changes in variables with more than two categories is not additive. Rather it is multiplicative and may be estimated by:

$$[(EXP\ (coefficient))^x - 1] \times 100 \qquad [7]$$

where EXP indicates that the coefficient is exponentiated; and
where, x equals the number of level changes

Inclusion of censored data. One of the advantages of EHA is that it permits the use of all data regardless of the length of follow-up. The characteristics for every subject who participates in a study may be included in computations. From the point in time that a subject is *not* tracked (due to the termination of the study, to dropout, to placement, etc.), she or he is considered "censored" and is eliminated from computations. But up to that point in time, all information about censored cases is included in the estimation of a hazard and its covariates. At the point of censoring, subjects are classified as "placed" or "missing" (depending on the case outcome). Thus, EHA makes maximum use of collected data. It is, in a sense, analogous to aggregate logit analyses of success and failure for each day of a study (during which, of course, the sample size varies due to censoring).

Censoring may be "left" or "right" and "unbiased" or "biased." While this is an important topic on which there is a growing body of research, a detailed discussion of censoring and testing for bias is beyond the scope and space limitations of this paper. For more information, see Allison (1984) and Blossfeld, Hamerle, and Mayer (1989).

Order of entry. For multivariate EHA, the order of entry for explanatory variables may be controlled as in OLS regression. In this report, we used a blockwise, forward approach which constrained the order of entry to the order that information becomes available to workers and program administrators during the course of IFPS. That is, we wanted to replicate the order that information is revealed to IFPS staff in practice. In determining eligibility and drawing up treatment plans at intake, IFPS staff often must make decisions on the basis of scant information regarding client demographic characteristics and presenting problems. The degree to which such information is correlated with subsequent outcomes might be particularly useful in creating intake guidelines and service standards. Thus the first block contained a large group of referral and intake characteristics followed by mean goal achievement and service characteristics. These were allowed to enter equations using a $p < .05$ two-tailed criterion, and only social, demographic, and FRS variables that were significantly related to the hazard function at the bivariate level were placed in the pool of variables eligible for inclusion.

Then, to account for changes that occurred during the course of treatment, FRS posttest variables were allowed to enter. For all posttest variables that entered the equations, the corresponding pretest variable–if it was not already in the model–was forced into the equation. Only with such a control for intake characteristics was an exit variable allowed to remain in an equation.

Readers are cautioned that this approach has an important limitation. Within each block, variables were entered on the basis of sample-specific criteria. Across samples, small perturbations in the variance-covariance matrix may alter the order of entry, producing different partitions, and resulting in quite different models. Because models are highly influenced by the order of entry, comparison of substantive findings across methods and samples may be confounded by minor changes in sample sizes, bivariate correlations, and standard errors. In light of this, the findings that we present later in this paper should be viewed as exploratory.

The proportionality assumption. The PH model has the advantage of requiring no laborious search for a hazard distribution that fits an observed hazard rate. But as discussed in [4], [5], and [6], it requires that the ratio of hazards be constant for any two individuals at any point in time. This is called proportionality.

Proportionality may be graphically portrayed using "log minus log" plots, and it may be tested statistically by creating a time interaction term (Hopkins, 1988). The log minus log transformation of the survival function is given by:

$$\ln [-\ln S_0(t)^{\exp(b'z)}] \qquad [8]$$

where, $S_0(t)$ is an estimate of the survivor function based on a vector of covariates.

When proportionality is violated, several different strategies may be adopted. First, if the data permit, a model that includes a variable thought to violate the assumption may be estimated using an independent computational method such as logistic regression or discriminant analysis. There is reason to believe that partial likelihood estimation is relatively robust against violations of proportionality (Allison, 1984), and the use of an alternative method of estimation may confirm a result based upon the inclusion of a variable that fails proportionality. Unfortunately, logistic regression and discriminant analysis do not make use of time in the way that EHA does and thus, with a dissimilar solution, one cannot be sure whether findings differ because proportionality is compromised in EHA or because the loss of time-related information significantly affects the logistic or discriminant model.

A second and common approach involves the stratification of the variable which fails proportionality. Computationally, stratification involves the estimation and aggregation of a model across the *j* categories of an explanatory variable. This controls for the stratified variable because parameters are estimated within and aggregated across strata or levels of a variable. One set of regression coefficients for the remaining covariates is produced. A coefficient is not estimated for the stratified variable.

Third, a model for each level of the explanatory variable that violates proportionality may be estimated. Analogous to stratification, this approach is rooted in the possibility that causal structures may be different for different levels of a covariate. As with stratification, this approach leads to models without a parameter estimate for the covariate that is the source of nonproportionality.

If the lack of such an estimate is problematic, a fourth approach may be worth investigation. The variable that violates proportionality may be recoded in such a way as to satisfy proportionality. The process of collapsing a continuous variable to a dummy variable plus the use of alternative estimation methods will be demonstrated in this paper.

Testing hypotheses. In order to test the hypothesis that the parameter estimates-that is, the regression coefficients for covariates-are not significantly different from zero, a likelihood ratio (LR) test is used. It takes the form of:

$$LR = 2[\ln L(B_{full\ model}) - \ln L(B_{restricted\ model})] \quad [9]$$

where lnL = the log likelihood of a model with or without covariates.

This test requires a large sample and has a chi-square distribution when the null hypothesis is true. Significance suggests that parameter estimates are significantly different from zero (Hopkins, 1988, p. 734; Blossfeld, Hamerle, & Mayer, 1989, p. 88).

FINDINGS

Of the 409 children, 92 (22.5%) were placed during the study period. During treatment, 25 children were placed, and during follow-up, the remaining 67 experienced at least one out-of-home episode of two weeks duration or more. The placement prevention rate at case termination was 93.9 (384/409) percent. Over the entire period, the placement prevention rate was 77.5 per cent.[1]

In Table 2, four alternative approaches to the estimation of the correlates of placement are shown. Column (A) shows an EHA proportional hazards solution with mean goal achievement computed as a summated scale. Column (C) shows an EHA proportional hazards solution with mean goal achievement computed as a binary variable. Using the same data set, logistic regression (E) and discriminant analysis (G) solutions are presented to demonstrate the results from the use of alternative methods of estimation. Sample sizes vary slightly because of missing data.

The Correlates of Placement

Substantively, the PH model findings (column A) suggest that ethnic/racial minority children had significantly lower risks of placement when a variety of intake, service, and family factors were controlled. The exponentiated value of the ethnic/racial minority coefficient (-.772) is .462, indicating that minority children were some 54% less likely to experience placement [(.462-1.0) × 100] when compared to other children (see [7]). In the same vein, teenagers were some 82% more likely to be placed than younger children [(exp .601-1.0) × 100], while children with at least one prior placement had a risk of placement that was 66%

Table 2
Comparative Estimates of Coefficients for Four Models of Placement in Washington

Variables	Proportional Hazards (A) Coeff	Proportional Hazards (B) t-value	Proportional Hazards (C) Coeff	Proportional Hazards (D) t-value	Logistic Regression (E) Coeff	Logistic Regression (F) t-value	Discriminant Analysis (G) Coeff	Discriminant Analysis (H) lambda
Intake Characteristics								
Primary caretaker's age							.041***	.939
Ethnic/racial minority	-.772*	-2.282	-.787*	-2.324	-1.341**	-2.921	-.307***	.873
At least one family member is employed							.287***	.846
Number of children at home	.601*	2.397	.571*	2.180			-.061***	.930
Child age 13 to 17 (teen)					1.241***	3.968	.220***	.884
Child has at least one prior placement	.506*	2.202	.514*	2.231	.746*	2.522	.222***	.862
Length of last placement (months)							.088***	.845
Child is at home at referral							-.097***	.858
Child is at home at intake	-.694*	-2.242	-.769*	-2.485			-.151***	.857
Child is truant at intake							.186**	.842
Child has drug/alcohol involvement at intake			.491*	2.090			.144***	.898
Treatment Goals								
Mean goal achievement	-.714***	-4.613	-1.574***	-4.850	-1.128*	-2.000	-.461***	.970
Concrete Services								
Time spent on concrete services							-.049***	.959
Social Support (Primary Caretaker)								
Coaching from extended family or other (at least twice a week)					1.115***	3.301		
Family Risk Scales								
Mental disturbance or illness of parent at intake	.736**	2.576					.241***	.920
Parent seems concerned but careless or indifferent about problems, rejects parental role at exit			.704*	2.436	1.396**	3.230		

146

Table 2, cont.
Comparative Estimates of Coefficients for Four Models of Placement in Washington

Variables	Proportional Hazards (A) Coeff	(B) t-value	(C) Coeff	(D) t-value	Logistic Regression (E) Coeff	(F) t-value	Discriminant Analysis (G) Coeff	(H) lambda
Parent prefers to place child (but willing to delay) or asks for immediate placement at intake	1.055***	4.043	1.091***	4.200	.808*	2.057		
Child's physical needs are met marginally or inadequately at intake			−.737*	−2.411				
Child's physical needs are met marginally or inadequately at exit[1]	−.683*	−1.792			−1.108*	−2.231		
Parent rarely demonstrates affection and may reject child openly at intake					.900**	2.647	.375***	.822
Log Likelihood	−441.267***		−441.547***					
−2 Log Likelihood					319.152++		72.259****	
Model Chi-Square					87.824***			
N	380		380		386		379	

Column (A) represents unstandardized coefficients of the PH model with continuous mean goal achievement.
Columns (B), (D), and (F) represent (coeff/standard error) for the models (A), (C), and (E).
Column (C) represents unstandardized coefficients of the PH model with discrete mean goal achievement.
Column (E) represents unstandardized coefficients of the logistic regression model.
Column (F) shows t-value of the logistic regression model.
Column (G) represents standardized canonical discriminant function coefficients of discriminant analysis.
Column (H) shows Wilks' lambdas of the discriminant analysis.
[1] An unshown control for the intake level of this variable was entered in the equation.
+ p<.10
* p<.05
** p<.01
*** p<.001
++ p=.980, df=373

higher than children who had no placement history [(exp .506–1.0) × 100]. A child whose primary caretaker was rated by workers as functioning poorly in the home because of mental illness or disturbance was more likely to be placed. And, similarly, children whose parents or caretakers requested placement at intake were more likely to be placed. Curiously, children whose parents inadequately or marginally met their physical needs (food, shelter, toys, etc.) were less likely to be placed. This appears to suggest that the lack of family resources by itself was not sufficient to produce placement in the sample.

Two factors act in a protective fashion and provide some preliminary clues as to what might account for the apparent success of IFPS. Children who were in their homes at intake had significantly higher success rates when compared to children who were not at home at the start of service. Children who were reunified with their parents shortly after intake or who, for other reasons, were not in the home at intake were approximately 50% more likely to experience a subsequent placement. While the reunification of families separated by placement is an alternative use of IFPS, it appears that successes equivalent to those observed in preventing placements among families where children are in the home at intake may not be found. Independent of prior placements, success is promoted when children are in the home–whether recently returned or not–at the start of service.

Second, mean goal achievement was correlated with service success. Although other factors appear to identify families that may be at greater risk of service failure, the relative strength of mean goal achievement suggests that, controlling for these factors, goal achievement exerts a significant influence on service outcomes. This may be an important finding, but, unfortunately, mean goal achievement did not meet the proportionality assumption.

A statistical test given by Kalbfleisch and Prentice (1980) and visual inspection of the log minus log transformation of the survival function [8], as shown in Figure 3, indicated that children from families with differing goal achievement scores had quite different survival profiles. Two log minus log plots are shown, each represents a different method of computing mean goal achievement. In the top plot (we will discuss the bottom plot later in the paper), mean goal achievement is computed using four levels. Mean goal achievement scores could range from 1.0 to 5.0. Scores were partitioned into four categories: A = 1-1.999; B = 2-2.999; C = 3-3.999; and D = 4-5.000. The X-axis, TIME, is shown in months but was measured and calculated in days. Visual inspection of this plot suggests that proportionality is not satisfied.

For each variable in the equation, an additional test was undertaken. This test of proportionality involved creating an interaction term between time and each explanatory measure. Comparable to the testing of interaction in OLS regression, this interaction term is entered in an equation and when its coefficient is significant, proportionality may be violated (Hopkins, 1988, pp. 726-728; Kalbfleisch & Prentice, 1980).

FIGURE 3

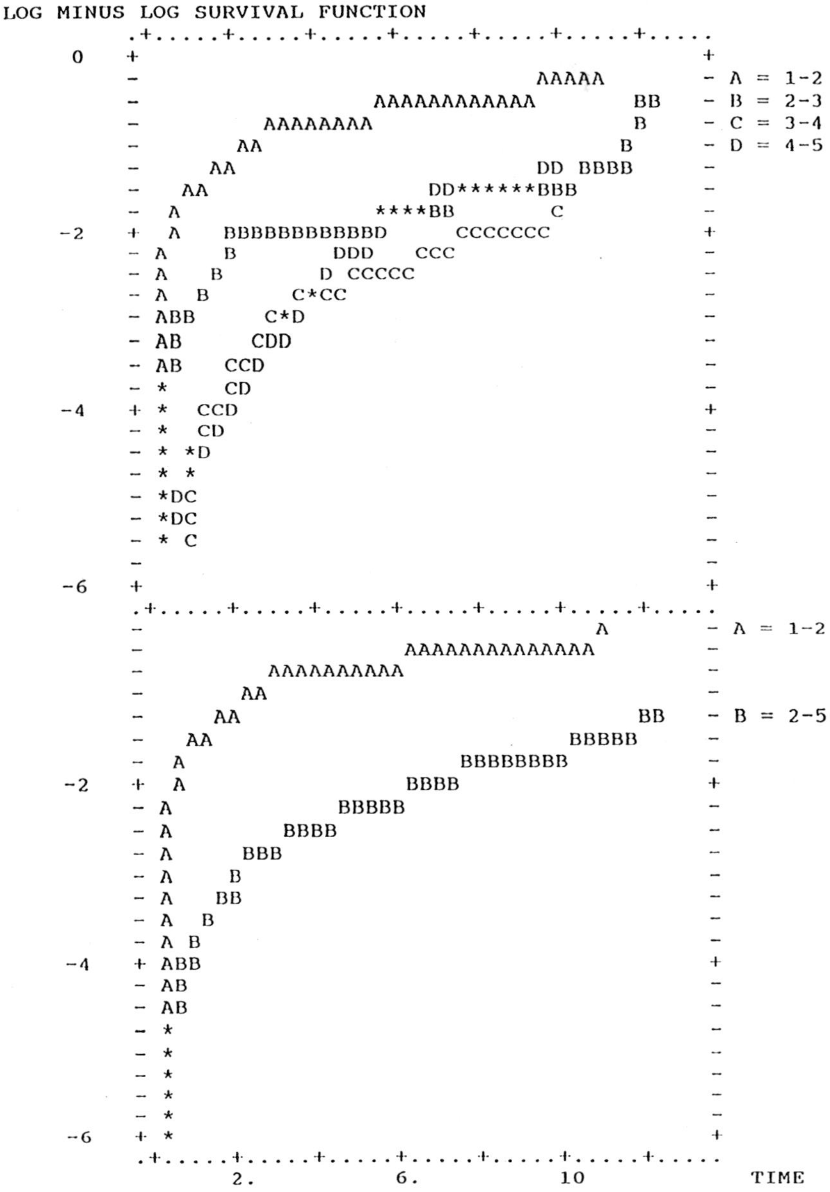

```
LOG MINUS LOG SURVIVAL FUNCTION
        .+.....+.....+.....+.....+.....+.....+.....
    0   +                                              +
        -                              AAAAA           -   A = 1-2
        -                   AAAAAAAAAAAA    BB         -   B = 2-3
        -            AAAAAAAA                B         -   C = 3-4
        -         AA                         B         -   D = 4-5
        -       AA                       DD BBBB       -
        -      AA                     DD******BBB      -
        -     A                  ****BB         C      -
   -2   +    A   BBBBBBBBBBBD      CCCCCCC             +
        -   A    B        DDD    CCC                   -
        -   A    B          D CCCCC                    -
        -   A  B        C*CC                           -
        -   ABB       C*D                              -
        -   AB       CDD                               -
        -   AB      CCD                                -
        -   *       CD                                 -
   -4   +  *     CCD                                   +
        -  *     CD                                    -
        -  *   *D                                      -
        -  *  *                                        -
        -  *DC                                         -
        -  *DC                                         -
        -  * C                                         -
        -                                              -
   -6   +                                              +
        .+.....+.....+.....+.....+.....+.....+.....
        -                                A             -   A = 1-2
        -                       AAAAAAAAAAAAAA         -
        -              AAAAAAAAAA                      -
        -           AA                                 -
        -         AA                           BB      -   B = 2-5
        -        AA                         BBBBB      -
        -       A                        BBBBBBBB      -
   -2   +      A                     BBBB              +
        -     A                   BBBBB                -
        -     A                BBBB                    -
        -     A             BBB                        -
        -     A        B                               -
        -     A       BB                               -
        -     A  B                                     -
        -     A B                                      -
   -4   +  ABB                                         +
        -   AB                                         -
        -   AB                                         -
        -   *                                          -
        -   *                                          -
        -   *                                          -
        -   *                                          -
        -   *                                          -
   -6   +  *                                           +
        .+.....+.....+.....+.....+.....+.....+.....
              2.        6.       10            TIME
```

We say "may" because Tuma (1990) has recently challenged the validity of the Kalbfleisch and Prentice statistical test, and thus it is not clear at present whether the interaction of time with a covariate can be used to assess proportionality. However, the visual inspection of log minus log plots continues to be an accepted and reasonable method by which to examine (at least, in a crude way) the proportionality of a variable. One is left, though, without a clear criterion for determining at what point survival plots which are not exactly parallel warrant the decision that proportionality is violated. More research is needed–and will undoubtedly be undertaken–on this issue.

Alternatives When Proportionality Is Violated

Because mean goal achievement is a variable for which a relative estimate of its effect would be useful (i.e., an understanding of its importance relative to the other correlates of placement), stratification and separate analysis by levels of achievement were not viewed as desirable alternatives. In this case, we wanted to estimate the effect of mean goal achievement in the context of the other correlates that emerged in PH model (A). Three alternatives are demonstrated below.

Discriminant analysis. Initially, a discriminant analysis model was estimated with a binary success-failure dependent measure. Shown in Table 2 (column G), the discriminant solution contained six of the eight variables in the PH (A) model. Teenage, ethnic-minority children who had more extensive placement histories and whose parents' capacity to perform child caring functions was impaired by mental illness were identified as at greater risk of placement. Further appearing to confirm the PH (A) model, children who were at home at the start of service were less likely to be placed, and service goal achievement significantly reduced the risk of placement.

Disconfirming the PH (A) model, however, parental preference for placement at intake and the degree to which children's needs were met at the close of service did not enter the model. Moreover, nine additional variables entered the discriminant solution. Older parents who were employed outside the home were more likely to have children who were placed subsequent to treatment intake. Larger families appear to have been at lower risk. Children who were truant, drug involved, and rejected by their parents were also found to be at greater risk of placement.

While the discriminant analysis contained much of the PH (A) findings, two PH (A) findings were not replicated and a suspicious array of additional correlates were identified. Further examination of the discriminant solution indicated that homoscedasticity across the success and failure groups may not have been satisfied. Box's M was significant (M = 317.81, p < .001) and visual inspection of the standard deviations for variables in the success-failure groups indicated that there was more variation in the success condition than in the failure condition. Thus, although the findings were rich and tempting, the statistical properties of the discriminant solution raised doubts about its validity.

Logistic regression. Using maximum likelihood logistic regression–a procedure that is more robust than discriminant analysis against heteroscedasticity–a second model with a binary dependent measure was then estimated. See Table 2, column E. Across six variables, this model was similar to the PH (A) model. The signs of the variables in the logistic solution were the same as the signs in the PH (A) solution, and mean goal achievement was significantly related to placement. The logistic findings lent support to the PH (A) solution.

Intriguingly, however, three new variables entered the logistic model. These variables were "coaching" of the primary caretaker by extended family members or others in the family's social network (a factor-based index), caretakers' attitudes toward the parenting role at the close of service, and parental demonstration of affection toward the child at intake. Substantively, each variable makes sense. For example, the parents of children who were more likely to be placed appear to have had more "coaching" from extended family members. When a family's problems spill over into public acknowledgment within the larger family, it usually indicates greater dysfunction. Families in which parents reported that relatives and others provided advice ("You ought to stop hitting Billy") and direction ("You need to get help") were more likely to fail in treatment. The presence of this kind of informal helping should signal IFPS workers that extra efforts may be necessary to protect children, but it also suggests that resources may be available within the social network that might be mobilized to help with child care and other family needs.

Although the variables were intuitively appealing, one must ask, why would three new variables enter the model? The answer lies, we think, in the nature of the dependent variable. In logistic regression and discriminant analysis, the occurrence of an event constitutes the outcome measure. In event history analysis, the occurrence of an event *plus* time constitute the outcome measure. Event history analysis makes use of more information. The addition of time in the construction of an outcome measure makes possible a more restrictive solution: one that includes the impact of time-to-placement as well as the mere occurrence of placement.

If a goal of intensive family preservation programs is to prevent placement, then there is a logical corollary:

> Placement should be prevented as quickly as possible and for as long a time as is possible.

If one wishes to estimate the correlates of service outcomes, then, by this corollary, a placement that occurs two days after the close of service should be weighted more heavily than a placement that occurs ten months distant from the close of service. Such a ten month placement is, many would think, far less likely to have been affected by service. Our point is that time cannot be ignored as a variable. And neither logistic regression nor discriminant analysis permit the differential weighting of cases on the basis of time-to-placement. Event history analysis does.

Cornering a nonproportional variable. A solution that uses EHA and produces an estimate of the impact of mean goal achievement was desirable. Short of stratification, an alterative that serves these objectives is to corner the variable which is the source of nonproportionality into categories that meet proportionality. By examining the log minus log plots (see [8]), it may be possible on occasion to create a cornered variable that meets proportionality. Although this sacrifices information, it was done, and mean goal achievement was collapsed into a binary variable such that: 0 to 2 = 0; and scores greater than 2 = 1. As shown in the log minus log plot in the bottom half of Figure 3, this new variable appears to satisfy proportionality and when used in PH (C), a model quite similar to PH (A) was produced.

This approach permitted a new estimate of the relationship between mean goal achievement and placement. Controlling for the other correlates of time-to-placement, children whose families were rated as achieving at least 25% of their goals (level 2 or more) were approximately 79% [exp-.1.574-1.0) × 100] less likely to be placed subsequent to service.

PH (C) and PH (A) are not statistically different, but one satisfies proportionality and the other does not. The likelihood ratio tests [9] are nearly identical and the substantive content of the models is similar. PH (C) suggests that children whose families were referred for neglect fared somewhat better in treatment. That is, children whose physical needs were marginally or inadequately met at intake were at a lower risk of placement. This is consistent with other findings (Fraser, Pecora, & Haapala, in press). Similar also to other findings, PH (C) suggests that children who had drug and alcohol involvement at intake were some 63% more likely to be placed than children referred for other reasons. On balance, then PH (C) appears both to replicate and extend PH (A).

Finally, we would like to briefly demonstrate a use of stratification. Shown in Table 3, a third "confirmatory" EHA model was estimated by stratifying goal achievement in PH (C), that is computing coefficient estimates for the covariates within the two categories of mean goal achievement and aggregating the results. With the exception that no coefficient for goal achievement was produced, the stratified solution replicated closely the PH (C) solution. For example, the coefficient for ethnic/minority in PH (C) was -.787 and in the stratified model it was -.777. For drug and alcohol involvement, the PH (C) coefficient was .491, while in the stratified model it was .511. For prior placement, the coefficient in PH (C) was .514, whereas in the stratified model it was .490. For parents' mental disturbance, it was .665 in the stratified model and .704 in PH (C). The largest difference was observed for child's physical needs at intake, where PH (C) was -.737 and the stratified model was -.671. On balance, stratification confirmed

Table 3

Estimated Event History Coefficients for Stratified Model of Placement in Washington

Variable	Coefficient	t-value
Intake Characteristics		
Ethnic/racial minority	-.777*	-2.293
Child age 13 to 17 (teen)	.573*	2.184
Child has at least one prior placement	.490*	2.129
Child is at home at intake	-.728*	-2.352
Child has drug/alcohol involvement at intake	.511*	2.166
Family Risk Scales		
Mental disturbance or illness of parent at intake	.665*	2.316
Parent prefers to place child (but willing to delay) or asks for immediate placement at intake	1.007***	3.824
Child's physical needs are met marginally or inadequately at intake	-.671*	-2.194
Log Likelihood	-411.826***	
N	380	

*p<.05.
***p<.001.

the PH (C) model. Thus, even when a coefficient for a nonproportional variable is desired, stratification may be used to confirm the remainder of a model.

DISCUSSION

Using event history analysis to build models of service success/failure, the findings suggest that families with teenage children who have more extensive histories of out-of-home placement and drug involvement are at greater risk of placement during and after treatment. The findings also imply that families where parenting is affected by mental illness or where parents have given up hope and requested placement have a higher risk of service failure.

Importantly, IFPS appears to be relatively more successful among ethnic and racial minority families. This finding bears careful examination, for only 18.3% of the sample were ethnic minorities and all ethnic/minority categories were collapsed for comparison to white, non-Hispanic families. It is likely that success varies across ethnic and racial minority groups, and future research with adequate samples of Black, Hispanic, Asian, and other minorities is needed. Historically, such findings have been a rarity in social welfare research. Because ethnic/racial minority children are known to be placed disproportionately out of their homes, IFPS programs based on the HOMEBUILDERS model may provide a viable alternative to the extensive use of substitute care for minority children.

Importantly also, modest goal achievement significantly increased a child's chances of remaining in her/his home. Future research might address the correlates of goal achievement, for goal achievement may mediate other risk factors (see Fraser, Pecora, & Haapala, in press). Such data would have utility in developing supplementary services for IFPS and in the creation of service standards.

From a methods perspective, the results demonstrate the potential of event history analysis in social welfare research. The use of methods that include only a dichotomous measure of the occurrence of an event appear to lead to slightly different models. This is especially the case when the assumptions of discriminant analysis are violated. Given the reliance of researchers in the field of family-based services on discriminant analysis, caution should be exercised in interpreting the findings of many recent studies.

Implications for the Collection of Event Data

To use event history analysis, we make several suggestions. First, use the smallest possible, reasonable unit of time. In much social research, days may be adequate, but in drug reaction research, for example, hours may be more precise. The unit of time should be sufficiently small to permit easy differentiation of early, mid, and late occurring events.

Second, collect data on precise times. Avoid rounding to the first of the month, heaping events on the last working day of the month, etc. EHA is sensitive to small differences and time data that load events on Fridays, holidays, and the like may produce invalid coefficient estimates.

Third, keep track of second, third, and other subsequent events. The causal structures for subsequent events may differ and you may want to undertake separate analyses for second or third events, given a first event.

Fourth, record data about previous events. The date of the most recent prior placement (or other event) may influence the date of the next placement, and in many studies it may be necessary to control for both the occurrence and date of prior events.

Fifth, become familiar with the distributional properties of your data. Exercise care when introducing skewed variables to equations. Our experience suggests that EHA can be sensitive to a few extreme cases. Outliers and nonlinearities must be carefully examined.

Sixth, while EHA appears to be robust against violations of proportionality, slightly different models may be produced when cornered variables are substituted for variables with a larger number of categories. Stratify cornered, nonproportional variables to confirm the presence, direction, and significance of other variables in a model.

With regard to proportionality, there are no fully accepted criteria for determining nonproportionality and thus it makes sense to make maximum use of graphical techniques, alternative methods, separate estimation for levels of variables that fail proportionality, stratification, and cornering to rescale problematic variables. Finally, at present, there are no algorithms for EHA that are fully comparable to r-square, and thus the degree to which EHA models account for variation in hazards cannot be estimated.

Event history analysis is a new and evolving statistical technique. Its sensitivities are only now being discovered and procedures to adjust for them are only now being developed. A substantial literature, for example, has been generated on the effects of unobserved heterogeneity on coefficient estimates (see Blossfeld & Hamerle, 1988; Trussell & Richards, 1985; Tuma & Hannan, 1984; Yamaguchi, 1986). And even simple measurement error-error uncorrelated with any particular explanatory variable-may bias parameter estimates (Tuma, forthcoming). Caution is warranted. Notwithstanding, while EHA cannot be used without careful analyses of bivariate hazard rates and tests for violations of basic assumptions, it appears to provide social work researchers with a powerful new tool for the estimation of structural models with time varying dependent and explanatory measures.

REFERENCES

Allison, P. D. (1984). *Event history analysis: Regression for longitudinal event data*. Beverly Hills, CA: Sage Publications.

Allison, P. D. (1988). *Event history analysis*. Philadelphia, PA: University of Pennsylvania.

AuClaire, P., & Schwartz, I. M. (1986). *An evaluation of the effectiveness of intensive home-based services as an alternative to placement for children and their families.* Minneapolis, MN: Hennepin County Human Service Department & the University of Minnesota, Hubert H. Humphrey Institute of Public Affairs.

Bienen, H., & Van De Walle, N. (1989). Time and power in Africa. *American Political Science Review, 83*(1), 19-34.

Blossfeld, H., & Hamerle, A. (1988). Unobserved heterogeneity in hazard rate models: A test and an illustration from a study of career mobility. In K. U. Mayer & N. B. Tuma (Eds.), *Event histories analysis in life course research.* Madison, WI: University of Wisconsin Press.

Blossfeld, H., Hamerle, A., & Mayer, K. U. (1989). *Event history analysis.* Hillsdale, NJ: Lawrence Erlbaum Associates.

Callister, J. P., Mitchell, L., & Tolley, G. (1986). Profiling family preservation efforts in Utah. *Children Today, 15,* 23-25, 36-37.

Campbell, R. T., Mutran, E., & Parker, R. N. (1986). Longitudinal design and longitudinal analysis: A comparison of three approaches. *Research on Aging, 8*(4), 480-504.

Compher, J. V. (1983). Home services to families to prevent child placement. *Social Work, 28,* 360-364.

Cox, D. R. (1972). Regression models and life tables. *Journal of the Royal Statistical Society,* Series B, *34,* 187-202.

Cox, D. R. (1975). Partial likelihood. *Biometrika, 62*(2), 269-276.

Dixon, W. J., Brown, M. B., Engelman, L., Hill, M. A., & Jennrich, R. I. (Eds.). (1988). *BMDP statistical software manual* (Vol. 2). Berkeley, CA: University of California Press.

Edna McConnell Clark Foundation (1985). *Keeping families together: A case for family preservation.* New York: Author.

Fixsen, D. L., Olivier, K. A., & Blase, K. A. (1989). What to do after they open the door: Alberta family support services. Paper presented at the Empowering Families Conference, Third Annual Meeting of the National Association for Family-Based Services, Riverdale, IL.

Frankel, H. (1988). Family-centered, home-based services in child protection: A review of the research. *Social Services Review, 62,* 137-157.

Fraser, M. W., Pecora P. J., & Haapala, D. A. (1989). *Families in crisis: Findings from the family-based intensive treatment project.* Salt Lake City, UT: University of Utah, Graduate School of Social Work, Social Research Institute and Federal Way, WA: Behavioral Sciences Institute.

Fraser, M. W., Pecora, P. J., & Haapala, D. A. (in press). *Family-based intensive treatment: The impact of family preservation services.* New York, NY: Aldine de Gruyter.

Geismar, L., & Ayers, B. (1958). *Families in trouble.* St. Paul, MN: Family-Centered Project.

Haapala, D. A., & Kinney, J. M. (1988). Avoiding out-of-home placement of high-risk status offenders through the use of intensive home-based family preservation services. *Criminal Justice and Behavior, 15*(3), 334-348.

Hinckley, E. C., & Ellis, W. F. (1985). An effective alternative to residential placement: Home-based services. *Journal of Clinical Child Psychology, 14*(3), 209-213.

Hopkins, A. (1988). Survival analysis with covariates-Cox models. In W. J. Dixon, M. B. Brown, L. Engelman, M. A. Hill, & R. I. Jennrich (Eds.), *BMDP Statistical Software Manual, Volume 2*. Berkeley, CA: University of California Press.

Horejsi, C. R. (1981). The St. Paul family-centered project revisited: Exploring an old gold mine. In M. Bryce and J. C. Lloyd (Eds.) *Treating families in the home: An alternative to placement*. Springfield, IL: Charles C Thomas Publisher.

Jones, M. A. (1985). *A second chance for families: Five years later*. New York: Child Welfare League of America, 19-42.

Jones, M. A., Newman, R., & Shyne, A. W. (1976). *A second chance for families: Evaluation of a program to reduce foster care*. Washington, DC: Child Welfare League of America.

Jones, M. A., Magura, S., & Shyne, A. W. (1981). Effective practice with families in protective and preventive services: What works? *Child Welfare, 60*(2), 67-80.

Kalbfleisch, J. D., & Prentice, R. L. (1980). *The statistical analysis of failure time data*. New York, NY: John Wiley & Sons.

Kinney, J. M., Haapala, D. A., Booth, C., & Leavitt, S. (1990). Family-based practice: The evolution of the Homebuilder model. In J. K. Whittaker, J. Kinney, E. Tracy, and C. Booth (Eds.), *Reaching high risk families: Intensive family preservation in human services*. New York, NY: Aldine.

Kinney, J., Haapala, D., Booth, C., & Leavitt, S. (in press). *HOMEBUILDERS: Keeping families together*. Hawthorne, NY: Aldine de Gruyter.

Kinney, J. M., Madsen, B., Fleming, T., & Haapala, D. (1977). HOMEBUILDERS: Keeping families together. *Journal of Consulting and Clinical Psychology, 45*, 667-673.

Lawless, J. F. (1982). *Statistical models and methods for lifetime data*. New York, NY: John Wiley & Sons.

Magura, S. (1981). Are services to prevent foster care really effective? *Children and Youth Services Review, 3*, 193-212.

Magura, S., & Moses, B. S. (1986). *Outcome measures for child welfare services*. Washington, DC: Child Welfare League of America.

Magura, S., Moses, B. S., & Jones, M. A. (1987). *Assessing risk and measuring change in families: The family risk scales*. Washington, DC: Child Welfare League of America.

Nelson, K. E. (1990). Family-based services for juvenile offenders. *Children and Youth Services Review, 12*, 193-212.

Nelson, K. E., & Associates (1988). *Family based services: A national perspective on success and failure.* Iowa City, IA: National Resource Center on Family Based Services.

Pine, B. A. (1986). Child welfare reform and the political process. *Social Service Review, 60,* 339-359.

Rzepnicki, T. L. (1987). Recidivism of foster children returned to their own homes: A review and new directions for research. *Social Service Review, 61,* 56-70.

Slonim-Nevo, V., & Clark, V. A. (1989). An illustration of survival analysis: Factors affecting contraceptive discontinuation among American teenagers. *Social Work Research and Abstracts, 25*(2), 7-14.

Stein, T. J. (1985). Projects to prevent out-of-home placement. *Children and Youth Services Review, 7,* 109-122.

Trussell, J., & Richards, T. (1985). Correcting for unobserved heterogeneity in hazard models using the Heckman-Singer procedure. In N. B. Tuma (Ed.), *Sociological Methodological, 1985* (pp. 242-276). San Francisco, CA: Jossey-Bass.

Tuma, N. B. (forthcoming). Event history analysis: An introduction. In A. Dale & R. Davies (Eds.), *Analyzing social and political change: A casebook of methods.* Newbury Park, CA: Sage.

Tuma, N. B., & Hannan, M. T. (1984). *Social dynamics: Models and methods.* Orlando, FL: Academic Press.

Tuma, N. (1990). Event history analysis. Presentation at the Annual Meeting of the American Sociological Association.

Whittaker, J. K., Kinney, J., Tracy, E., & Booth, C. (Eds.), *Reaching high risk families: Intensive family preservation in human services.* New York, NY: Aldine.

Yamaguchi, K. (1986). Alternative approaches to unobserved heterogeneity in the analysis of repeatable events. In N. B. Tuma (Ed.), *Sociological Methodology, 1986* (pp. 213-219). San Francisco, CA: Jossey-Bass.

Yuan, Y. Y., & Associates (1990). *Evaluation of AB 1562 in-home care demonstration projects.* Sacramento, CA: Walter R. McDonald and Associates.

Moderator Variables in Social Work Research

Gary F. Koeske

SUMMARY. Moderator variables are "third variables" that affect the size or nature of the relationship between an independent and dependent variable. Because of this role, such expressions as specification, contingency, conditional, and qualification have been used in reference to moderator variables. In classical experimental research in psychology, moderator variables have been referred to as involved in "interaction effects" with the independent variable. Considering their important role in specifying under what conditions and for what subgroups variables will have significant effects, surprisingly little attention has been awarded moderator variables in social work research. This paper reviews the history of moderator variable applications in the related disciplines and exemplifies recent applications in the study of gender discrimination and research on stress, strain, and social support. Special attention is given to the comparison of correlations and slopes, factorial analysis of variance, and moderated regression analysis, since these are the dominant analytic strategies for detection and valuation of moderated effects. Less prominent procedures and refinements are briefly presented, as is the important role of moderator variables in theory explication and causal inference.

Much of contemporary social work research examines relationships among three or more variables. Analyses incorporated in this research have served to

---

Gary F. Koeske received his PhD in Social Psychology from Northwestern University. He is presently Associate Professor of Social Work at the University of Pittsburgh. His current research involves the study of stress and social support in work, school, and parenting environments. Recent publications relevant to the operation of moderated effects include: Koeske, G.F. and Koeske, R.D. (1990). The buffering effect of social support on parental stress. *American Journal of Orthopsychiatry, 60* (3), 440-451; Koeske, G.F. and Koeske, R.D. (1989). Workload and burnout: Can social support and perceived accomplishment help? *Social Work, 34* (3), 243-248.

This paper is a revision of a paper read at the annual convention of the Council of Social Work Education.

© 1992 by The Haworth Press, Inc. All rights reserved.

evaluate the impact of multiple potential causes, control for potentially extraneous variables, and elaborate intervening processes. Relatively little attention has been given to the incorporation of moderator variables. A moderator variable is any "third variable" over which a bivariate relationship is not general. Though "moderator" has become the most common term to describe such variable operation, specifier, qualifier, conditional, and contingent variable are also used. The process involved when a third variable qualifies a relationship is an "interaction effect." Such process terms as joint effect or multiplicative effect are frequently used as well. In the process terminology, the moderator variable (basically, a second independent variable) interacts with an independent variable in its effect on a dependent variable. Historically, interaction effects were mostly studied by experimental psychologists, but *moderator* (or specifier, qualifier) variables were examined by correlational researchers in psychology and sociology.

The term "moderator" arises from measurement applications in a decades-old psychology literature. In that tradition, moderator variables were typically subject characteristics that identified individuals for whom prediction equations worked differentially well (see Zedeck, 1971; Ghiselli, 1963). In effect, they were subject traits correlated with the error term in prediction equations. Present interest in moderator variables extends well beyond this historical use. They are now interesting to theoretically-oriented researchers who acknowledge and try to map the complexity of relationships. And, they are important for applied researchers attempting to achieve successful interventions by targeting programs to appropriate groups and environments.

MODERATOR VARIABLES AND EXTERNAL VALIDITY

One perspective on moderator variables is their relevance to the validity of conclusions drawn from an empirically noted relationship (see Cook & Campbell, 1979, for review of types of validity). There are four different threats to the inference that an X causes a Y. First, the X-Y relationship may be attributed to sampling variability, i.e., it may be a statistical fluke, a chance effect. Or, the X-Y relationship might be accounted for by reference to a potentially extraneous variable that is confounded with X. This second threat concerns *internal* validity. A third type of threat (experimental *construct* invalidity) arises when the mechanism or intervening variable presumed to be set in operation by the X stimulus is not the actual effective variable. The last threat to validity arises not from the operation of extraneous or intervening variables, but from moderator variables. A genuine impact of X on Y demonstrated in one context or for one group may not generalize to a different context or group. This is, of course, one issue in Campbell's familiar *"external validity."* So, we see that each of the three roles that third variables might play (extraneous, intervening, moderator) corresponds to one of the classical validity threats (internal, construct, and external, respectively).

Social workers and social work researchers have always been quite concerned with external validity, largely due to their concern with the effective application of findings. Applied researchers grant, of course, the need to acquire persuasive internal validity. Attention to establishing causation, however, often dictates highly-controlled experimental designs, resulting in findings that may apply only in artificial or limited environments, or for individuals quite different from those who need to be served. Experimental construct validity pertains to the (theoretical) mechanisms responsible for causal relationships. These mechanisms have not typically been a primary concern of applied researchers, perhaps regrettably, since they might frequently inform practice. Consequently, of the three threat categories, it is external validity which has chiefly concerned social work researchers. *It is ironic, then, that so little attention has been given to the prediction, detection, or interpretation of moderated effects in social work research.*

The Point in the Research Process in Which Qualification Occurs

Throughout the discipline of psychology in the last 30 or 40 years, research efforts have assessed the joint impact of two or more independent variables on a dependent variable. Typically these models have been statistically evaluated using factorial analysis of variance. Often the "second" independent variable was a subject status variable, such as gender or groupings based on a personality trait. Such "treatments by levels" designs populated the pages of some psychology journals. There were also many applications in which two independent variables were simultaneously manipulated, often with *a priori* predictions of a joint effect. When the second independent variable is a subject status variable, it is regarded as the moderator that may qualify the effect of the primary X on the outcome; when both independent variables are manipulated, which one is regarded as the moderator depends on the guiding theory or statistical convenience. Treatment by levels designs are correctly regarded as experimental studies, but caution must be taken to interpret main effects of a levels variable as correlated rather than experimental effects.

A significant treatment by levels interaction basically demonstrates constraint on the generality of the experimental treatment effect. This is a limitation of the bounds of applicability of an intervention, but if predicted by theory it is a useful expression of modesty. In fact, in this research context, the demonstration of predicted interaction effects is highly regarded as evidence of complex and refined theorizing, of a more mature and successful science. And, from the standpoint of application such research successes increase the likelihood that eventual helping interventions will be successful, because they are directed to appropriate persons and environments.

Sometimes moderator variables do not enter the investigative process until a main or general effect has been disconfirmed. Then the researcher may initiate a search procedure for conditions under which the initially-predicted effect is found. In such an "internal analysis" the data set is broken down *post hoc* into subgroups. Possibly the predicted effect can be demonstrated for one or more subgroups. On some occasions, the breakdown is done on the basis of some evidence that the experimental treatment has "taken" for only some of the subjects; the data are then reanalyzed exclusively for these impacted cases.

The timing of entry of a moderator effect is not a trivial issue. Predicted interactions suggest mature, refined theorizing. *Post hoc* (unanticipated) interactions may suggest a thoughtfulness regarding one's data, and a concern about improving theory and its application. Unpredicted moderator effects must be regarded, however, with some suspicion. Their operation must be replicated in an independent data set. Creative researchers can make *post hoc* sense out of nearly any configuration of data. The less well-articulated or flaccid the guiding theory, the more easily it may incorporate the qualification.

In an unknown number of cases, the situation is much more problematic. A researcher hard-pressed to show a predicted effect may review a number of moderator variable candidates, proceeding until one is found for which an interaction with the treatment occurs. It is not necessarily wrong to conduct such fishing expeditions. It is, though, incumbent on the researcher to report that they have occurred, how many fish were thrown back, and conclude that replication is required. When we find that many breakdowns have occurred and reported interactions resist even *post hoc* theoretical interpretation, we should place very little stock in reported interactions. In program evaluation applications reporting benefits for only unanticipated subgroups of clients, the research consumer is advised to treat the report as an *exploratory* investigation.

The Form and Nature of Moderated Effects: Types of Interactions

Interactions occur whenever the effect of one variable depends on the level of another variable. The form, nature, analysis, and meaning of an interaction depend on a number of considerations, including the way in which the variables are measured and the presence (or absence) of direct relationships of the moderator (Z) with either X or Y. The X, Y, and Z variables may be measured qualitatively (as two or more levels or groupings) or quantitatively, as score variables. For most of my examples, we will assume a dichotomous moderator and a continuous score for Y. The X variable may be dichotomous, polychotomous, or continuous, depending on the example.

Table 1 shows graphic representations of common interaction effects for which X and Y are score variables and Z is a dichotomy. In Case I, we see that the relationship of X and Y is opposite in sign at levels A and B of variable Z. Case II shows the case in which a non-zero relationship of X with Y occurs at one level of Z, but not at the other, i.e., an impact of X on Y is limited to only some

Table 1.
Common Interaction Situations

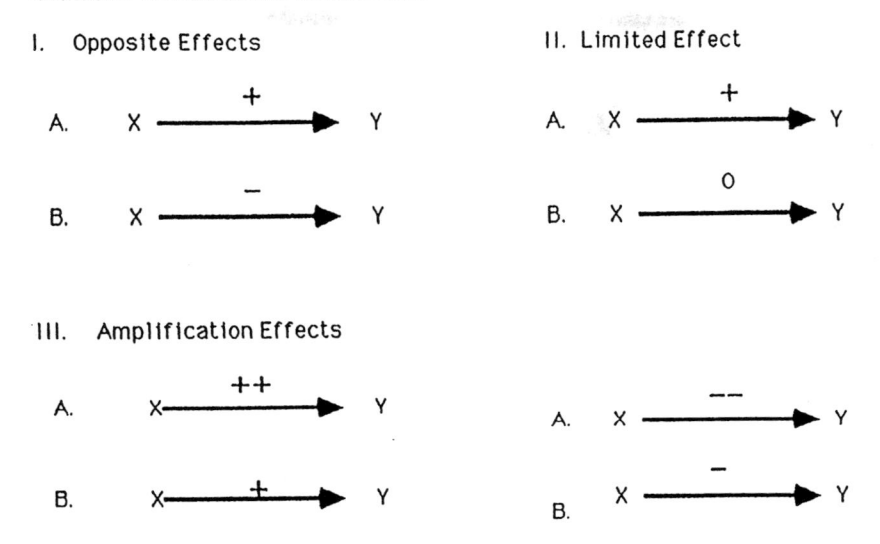

I. Opposite Effects

A. $X \xrightarrow{+} Y$

B. $X \xrightarrow{-} Y$

II. Limited Effect

A. $X \xrightarrow{+} Y$

B. $X \xrightarrow{0} Y$

III. Amplification Effects

A. $X \xrightarrow{++} Y$

B. $X \xrightarrow{+} Y$

A. $X \xrightarrow{--} Y$

B. $X \xrightarrow{-} Y$

conditions of Z. Case III shows an amplification-type interaction in which the impact of X on Y is significantly greater at one level of Z than at the other. These are the simplest possible interaction situations. When more than a single moderator is present (Z_1, Z_2, etc.), analysis and interpretation may become exceedingly complicated.

It is important to keep the effect of a variable on an X-Y relationship (the moderating effect) separate from whatever additional relationship the moderator may have to either X or Y. Frequently, variables of interest for their moderating quality may also be sensibly related to X and Y. We can easily see that this might be the case when variables such as gender and social support qualify the interrelationship of two other variables. Theory suggests that social support may "buffer" the impact of stress events on physical and mental health. That is, stress may impair health only for those lacking adequate social support (a Case II interaction in Table 1). In addition, those lacking social support may be independently more at risk for health problems–a direct effect of Z on Y. And, as a further complication in many research settings, social support may relate (in either a statistically positive or inverse manner) to the amount of stress experienced. Similarly, gender, as an early-established status variable, may moderate many empirical relationships, as well as relate directly to almost any X and Y.

In experimental applications, equal cell sizes assure that X and Z will be completely unrelated. When subjects drop out of the experiment, or when naturalistic groupings are employed, X and Z will typically be associated to some degree, perhaps highly associated in the latter case. This complicates statistical analyses, and solutions are controversial, although some are satisfactory to many practicing researchers. Finally, analysis and interpretation are more complicated when X and Z are polychotomous, rather than dichotomies or scores.

Moderator Variables and Causal Inference

An infrequently mentioned benefit of assessing moderator variables in hypothesis-testing correlational research is that it may facilitate a stronger inference of causal direction than when only X and Y are measured. In other words, predicting that an X-Y relationship will occur under one level of Z, but not under another, may be compatible *only* with the notion that X causes Y. It may not be derivable from the alternate directional interpretation that Y causes X. Without consideration of the moderator variable, the empirical correlation might be equally explicable as evidence for $Y \rightarrow X$ as $X \rightarrow Y$.

For example, a researcher might be able to conduct only a simple one-shot study in which measures of job satisfaction and life satisfaction are obtained for a sample of workers. The data might show a clearly significant correlation of job with life satisfaction. But this correlation would not uniquely support a theory that job satisfaction impacts on life satisfaction. If the researcher, however, had predicted that the correlation would be substantially higher (and perhaps only significant) for workers who had been employed for more than five years, the job→life satisfaction directional interpretation and corresponding theory would be meaningfully supported. The guiding presumption is that nothing inherent in the theory that life satisfaction causes job satisfaction would suggest the predicted qualification by number of years of employment, the moderator variable.

Further demonstration of how plausible inferences about causation can be made in correlational survey research through the explication and utilization of moderated effects (conditional relationships) can be found in Rosenberg's (1968) classic, *The Logic of Survey Analysis*. He summarizes several substantive examples by noting, "Conditional relationships may then provide a more complete causal analysis by stipulating the necessary conditions under which the determinative factors make their effects felt" (p. 145). The present emphasis differs from Rosenberg's in at least one important respect. His examples chiefly show how an incidentally-discovered conditional relationship may enhance theoretical and causal interpretation. The present suggestion is that researchers consciously incorporate moderated predictions into their models and thereby, given confirmation, strengthen the plausibility of *a priori* causal hypotheses in survey/correlational research. A published example of the use of a moderator variable to facilitate causal inference in correlational research can be found in Koeske and Koeske (1975).

Intervening Variables and Moderator Variables

The interpretation-clarifying role of postulating moderated effects can also be understood by consideration of the relationship between moderator variables and the mechanisms presumed to explain why X should impact on Y. When a particular Z variable is thought to qualify an X-Y relationship a process or mechanism is implicit. Let's say that we find that physical punishment discipline of young boys is associated with greater aggressiveness in adolescence. For girls, however, the relationship is reversed–much use of physical punishment is associated with less aggressiveness. The qualification of the discipline-aggressiveness relationship by gender suggests different theoretical mechanisms are operating for boys and girls. We might posit that due to sex role socialization, physical punishment procedures frustration and anger (the intervening variable) in males, but passivity/withdrawal in girls. So, different intervening mechanisms are required to explain the differing form of the relationships for boys and girls.

Similarly, if poverty is associated with high crime rates only when population density is high, we would be inclined to think in terms of mediators like "social constriction" and "invasion of personal space." Different theoretical constructs (mediators) would be needed to explain crime occurrences when poverty and density were not present jointly. Moderators and theoretical mechanisms work together in explanatory systems or models. Causal systems are enhanced by specifying the conditions necessary for relationships to occur in a postulated form. The benefit derived for causal inference mentioned above is simply a special case of the advantages derived from research being guided by carefully-articulated theories of social and behavioral process.

An awareness of the distinction between *moderated* and *mediated* relationships, and how the two processes work together to enrich complex causal modelling, has become the object of attention in the research community (ch. Baron & Kenny, 1986; Jaccard, Turrisi, & Wan, 1990). In the special case that a mediating process is measured (albeit indirectly), the researcher can carry out a more refined analysis of the operation of a theoretical moderator of the X-Y relationship. Consider, for example, the social support buffering notion mentioned earlier. Figure 1 presents results from Koeske and Koeske's (1990) burnout study in which Worker Stress stimuli were shown to affect Intention to Quit the job through their impact on Emotional Exhaustion (burnout). Social Support and a sense of Personal Accomplishment were hypothesized to moderate this stress-outcome relationship. That is, it was thought that stress elevated intention to quit primarily for workers lacking good social support and a sense of accomplishment in their work. Specifying the intervening variable of Emotional Exhaustion permitted evaluation of the moderating effects at each of two time points in the process. The figure shows that the *stress to exhaustion* relationship was not significantly qualified by the predicted moderators, but the *exhaustion to quitting* relationship was significantly qualified by both moderators. Exhaustion

FIGURE 1. Model of Moderating Effects of Social Support and Personal Accomplishment on Emotional Exhaustion and Intent to Quit

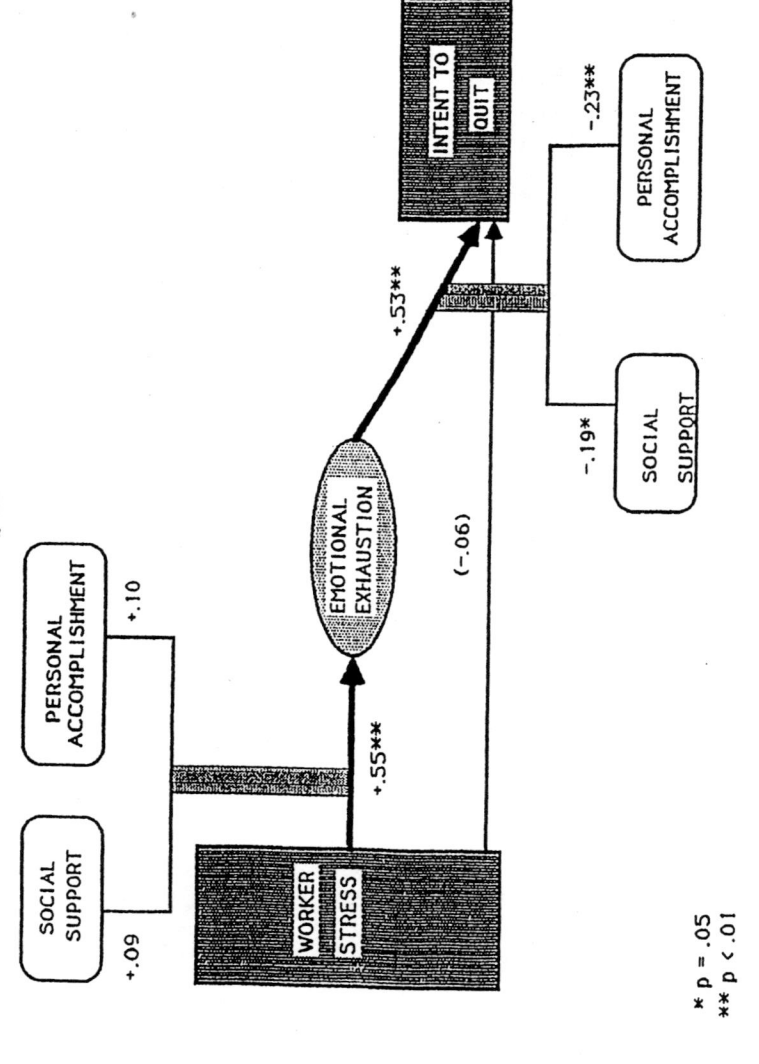

* p = .05
** p < .01

NOTES: PERSONAL ACCOMPLISHMENT coded so that high scores reflect felt efficacy with clients; Direct effects (in parentheses) predicted to be nonsignificant

resulted in intention to quit primarily for low support and low accomplishment workers.

These results suggest that stress may induce worker exhaustion regardless of favorable internal or external resources, but these resources may enable exhausted workers to sustain, endure, or cope with their work. Although the primary objective of this example is to delineate the advantages for theory and prediction of building models with moderator variables, the results have practical implications as well. They may suggest where in a dysfunctional process intervention can be most beneficial, and where it may be of little aid. For example, enhancing workers social support systems would seem to facilitate retention for workers experiencing what might be inevitable burnout; the same intervention may not effectively reduce the probability that exhaustion will arise in stressful work environments.

Analysis Schemes for Detecting and Evaluating Moderated Effects

The choice of an analytic scheme for testing or revealing interaction effects depends largely on how the X, Y, and moderator variables are measured. Other factors such as desired power, available sample size, expected nature of functional relationships, available software, and sophistication level of audience may also be considerations. Log linear analysis and logistic regression are available for applications in which the Y measure is a grouping variable (see Fienberg, 1977 for statistical content, and Wuthnow, 1978 for an interesting application), and structural equation (e.g., LISREL) solutions are in an early developmental stage (Kenny & Judd, 1984; Jaccard et al., 1990). Because very few published applications involve grouping dependent variables or adaptations of latent variable and structural equations analysis, this paper will focus on the most prevalent strategies used by social researchers.

Comparing correlations. Perhaps the simplest application involves comparing Pearson correlations of continuous X and Y variables (for examples, see Cooley & Keesey, 1981; Orpen, 1982). These correlations are obtained for two or more subgroups that define different levels of the Z (moderator) variable. A Fisher Z test for comparing two independent correlations (or a Chi Square test for comparing three or more correlations) could be conducted to determine if the size of the X→Y relationship was different for levels of the moderator variable.

As an example, we might consider the bivariate correlation on Number of Years of Education (X) with Income (Y). Education might be considered a merit variable that should increase income in a just world. Gender is a potential moderator of interest. In a non-discriminatory environment, it might be felt that education should be as highly correlated with income for women as for men. If the correlation for women were significantly lower than for men, we could infer that women were not being rewarded for a relevant merit factor-that discrimination occurred. Yamatani and Koeske (1984) tried to demonstrate that casting sex in the role of a moderator variable relative to merit-salary correlations could reveal evidence of discrimination obscured in classical detection schemes.

Comparing correlations, however, can be a seriously flawed practice. Let's say that we find a substantially higher correlation of education and income for male (.91) than female (.57) workers. Inferring that we had found evidence for sex discrimination would, however, be unacceptable. The evidence for gender as a moderator variable would be spurious, as shown in Figure 2 for hypothetical data (Set 1) from 12 male and 12 female workers. What we see is that the slopes of the regression lines for males (0.947) and females (0.928) are nearly identical: any increase in education for females produces the same income elevation as it does for males. The form and function of the X-Y relationship is not different for males and females, so there is no interaction with gender. The correlation is markedly higher for males, because the error of prediction is much greater for females (6.12 v. 1.98). There is a sense, though, in which data like these might suggest possible discrimination. The fact that a merit factor accounts for less variability in income scores for females could reflect that other unmeasured variables affect females' income.

The primary point of the above example is that comparing correlations (or standardized regression coefficients) can be misleading as an exclusive basis for determining the presence v. absence of moderated effects. An even more dramatic case may be seen in a different set of data graphed in Figure 3 (Data Set 2). This figure shows a higher correlation of education and income for females (R^2 = .682 v. .483), seemingly showing a more than equitable reward for women. Yet the slope of the regression line for males (0.814) is substantially steeper than for females (.326), imparting just the opposite information.

The use of gender as a moderator variable is informative, but not conclusive. The inference context is so complex that a number of conceptual and analytic strategies must be initiated. For instance, even a steeper slope for females than males may be interpretable as reflecting discrimination. In such a case, it may be argued that females must exhibit effort (acquiring education) to achieve a benefit where males need not. Perhaps males are granted income benefits on an arbitrary basis, or simply because of tenure. Additional analyses would be needed to compare male and female incomes at particular education levels–a conventional analysis of covariance (ANCOVA, with education as the covariate) might be used to compare gender salaries. The ANCOVA alone supplies only a fallible and partial answer, since it raises its own interpretive perplexities (see Cook & Campbell, 1979; Judd & Kenny, 1981).

Therefore, it is the unstandardized or metric coefficient which reflects the form of the X-Y relationship and imparts information about moderation by a third variable. Correlations and standardized regression coefficients may be very misleading. Yet, they are secondarily informative, and they can be reliably consulted when score variabilities and measurement error in the dependent

FIGURE 2. Relationship between Education and Income for Males and Females Showing No Interaction Effect Despite Differences in Correlations

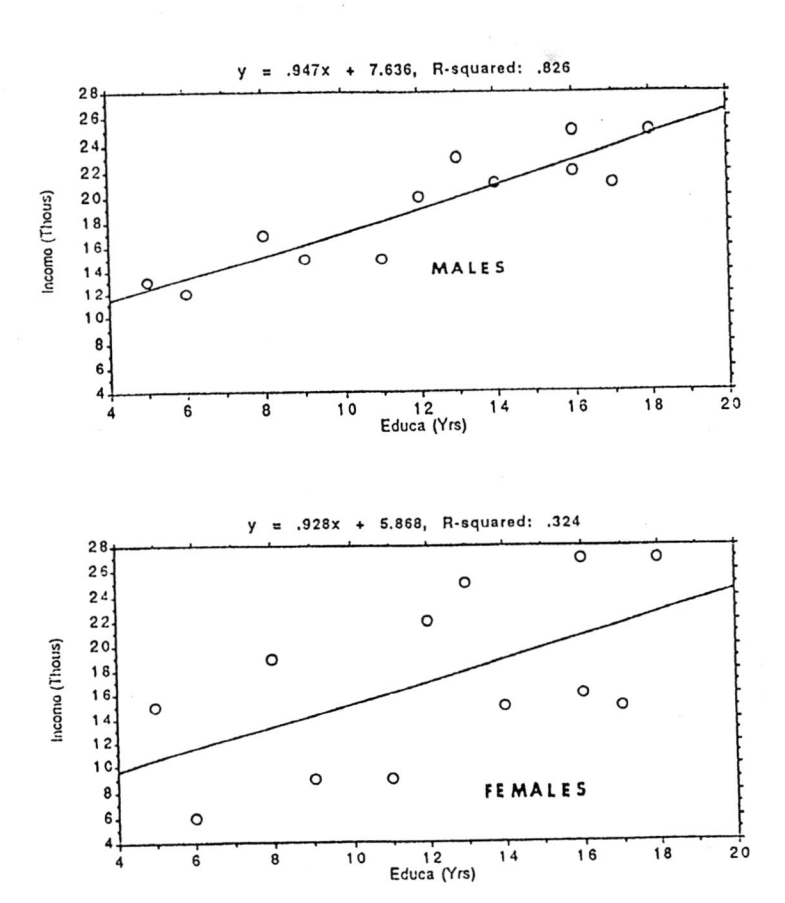

variable are not different between moderator variable levels. Jaccard et al. (1990) recommend that comparisons of correlations be limited to questions of same-versus-different validity coefficients, with non-standardized (metric) coefficients employed when inferences of causal relationship are the issue. Stone and Hollenback (1989, p. 8) argue that even tests of differential validity "may lead to erroneous conclusions about the importance of a suspected moderator variable," if they are based on a comparison of correlations.

FIGURE 3. Relationship between Education and Income Showing an Interaction Effect with a Higher Regression Coefficient for Males and a Higher Correlation Coefficient for Females

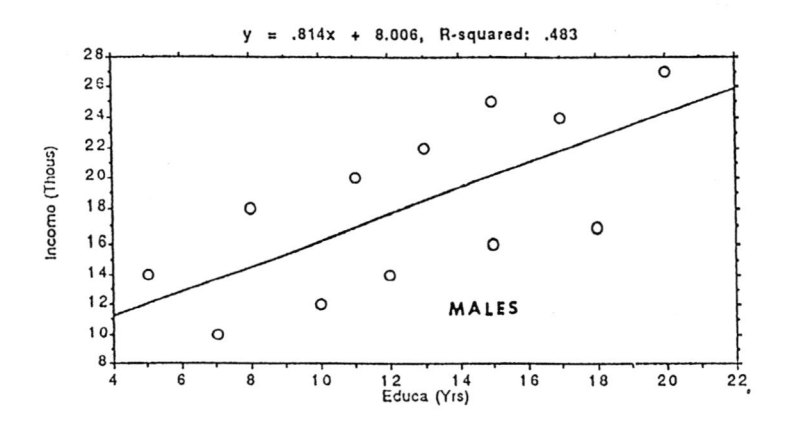

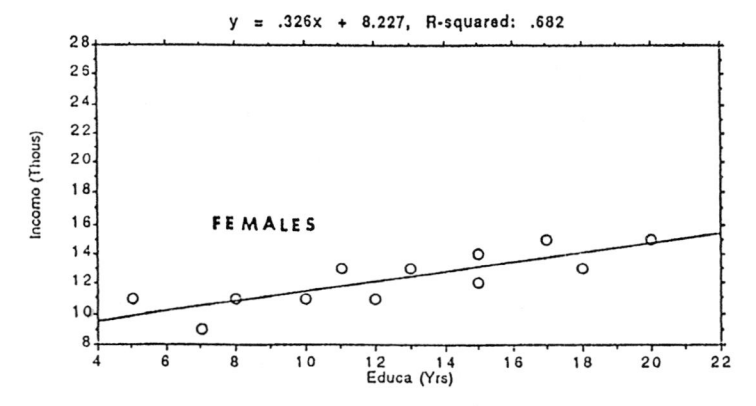

Analysis of variance (ANOVA). Although the expression "moderator variable" (Saunders, 1956) arose in a context in which continuous measures were employed, "interaction effects" were frequently examined in experimental research for which the independent and moderator variables were grouping variables. Interaction effects are assessed by an F test for the A X B (or higher order) interaction, and they are represented by A X B tables of means or by a plotting of these means on a graph. Whenever A and B are natural grouping variables (treatment group, sex, race, etc.) and Y is a score measure, factorial analysis of variance may be the most efficient and clear procedure for approaching interactions.

The ANOVA approach is quite efficient. In addition to providing a straightforward and comprehensive significance test for the interaction, it provides clear visual display in tabled means, and information about "main effects," i.e., the overall effects of gender and education across the levels of the other variable. One important liability, however, is the loss of precision in the measurement of a continuous variable such as Education, which must be debased to a categorical variable. A statistical comparison of slopes which retains all the information in Education as a continuous variable would probably be more powerful. In the case that X were an inherent grouping (say, nominal) variable, this relative disadvantage would not apply.

Factorial ANOVA has, however, limitations and complications in actual practice-ones that go beyond the usual parametric test requirements of homogenous variances and normal distributions. Usually a minor concern is that some ordinal interactions may be metric-bound and disappear if a monotonic transformation is performed on an original arbitrary metric (e.g., a square root transformation). Normally, such transformations would not be performed on socially-relevant behaviors. Yet, if cell n's were small, variances were heterogeneous, or distributions were severely non-normal, a transformation might be required. A more frequent problem is the occurrence of non-orthogonal, i.e., correlated, independent variables caused by unequal and disproportionate cell sizes. This problem may arise in true experimental contexts in which subjects have dropped out of conditions of the experiment, and it will nearly always occur when the independent variables are naturalistic or measured variables (e.g., in a study of the joint effect of three different parental discipline strategies and family SES on deviant behavior of adolescents).

In most applications by social work researchers, the X and Z variables would be to some extent interdependent. What is problematic in cases of correlated independent variables is not the estimate of the interaction because it is always assessed after the main effects have been subtracted out. It is the main effects that will be differently estimated, depending on whether the typical solution that assumes orthogonality or an alternate solution that adjusts for interdependence has been employed. Some authors (Tabachnick & Fidell, 1983) advise that the typical ("experimental") solution may be employed, if naturalistic independent variables correlate in the sample as they might be expected to in the population. Others advise some sort of means adjustment or a type of regression solution yielding unique sums of squares. Some researchers have employed power-crippling random dropping of cases from larger cells to avoid the problem.

Some statistical packages have default solutions that carry out a regression solution when cell sizes are unequal, others use the standard "experimental" solution that assumes orthogonality, unless the researcher elects an alternate option. Proportional cell frequencies (for which X and Z are correlated zero) are incorrectly analyzed by many packages, which introduce irrelevant corrections that underestimate main effects. Probably the best conservative recourse (in the typical situation confronting social researchers using factorial ANOVA with correlated independent and moderator variables) is a regression solution.

Another limitation of the factorial ANOVA is that it has low power for detecting ordinal interactions, such as those shown in Cases II and III of Table 1. In the case that there is a discernible slope (effect) for one condition, but not for another condition, ANOVA might yield a significant main effect for the primary independent variable, but no significant interaction. This may result even when the subgroup means are identical at one level of the moderator, and the entire main effect difference arises from a contrasting level. Bobko (1986) offered an analytic alternative, which was subsequently compared in a simulation study with factorial ANOVA and other corrective alternatives (Strube & Bobko, 1989). Each alternative to ANOVA employed planned orthogonal or non-orthogonal contrasts in some manner, and each possessed greater power for detecting a true interaction effect than factorial ANOVA. Koeske and Koeske (1991) recommend contrast analysis as one strategy for increasing the power of tests for the important buffering interaction of stress and social support, which, according to theory, possesses an ordinal form. An appropriate application of contrast analysis is superior to ANOVA (and to hierarchical regression analysis to be discussed later) when theory is available to direct the specification of contrasts.

The proper interpretation of interaction effects is another troubling issue confronting researchers. In 2 X 2 ANOVAs a significant interaction effect can usually be reliably interpreted by simple inspection of cell means. When there are more than 2 levels of either variable, however, it is often very difficult to draw statistically-defendable conclusions about the results. The conventional approach to this interpretive dilemma is to carry out a "simple effects" analysis in which the total sum of squares is repartitioned to permit a statistical evaluation of the effect of A separately within each level of B. Simple effects analysis, however, may not assist interpretation when the interaction is of the amplification ordinal variety (Case III in Table 1). In this situation, as Jaccard et al. (1990) have noted, the mean differences will be significant at each level of the moderator. In other words, from the significance test standpoint, an identical result is obtained for each level of the moderator. They discuss two alternatives to simple effects analysis: interaction comparisons and interaction contrasts. The former involves examination of a *series* of 2 X 2 ANOVAs, and the latter proposes use of orthogonal contrasts in an attempt to encompass the comparisons explicit in a predicted interaction.

Rosenthal and Rosnow (1985) recommend an alternative analytic procedure called "contrast analysis" for evaluating any type relationship discoverable from comparing subgroup means. They provide a generalization and clarification of the procedure of *planned orthogonal comparisons*. This is a very powerful approach for testing an interaction of a predicted form. For example, a specific buffering-type interaction of stress and social support on depression score means could be assessed by contrast analysis. This approach differs from the "interaction contrasts" mentioned by Jaccard et al. (1990) in that non-orthogonal contrasts might be required to efficiently evaluate the implications of a guiding theory. The use of the highly general Bonferroni inequality to hold the experiment-wise error rate at .05 for a set of orthogonal and non-orthogonal contrasts could be implemented as part of the contrast analysis. Rosenthal and Rubin (1984) and Jaccard et al. (1990) might be consulted for the logic and implementation of the Bonferroni inequality. *Contrast analysis would seem to have greater power than other contemporary statistical alternatives (including moderated regression analysis)*, unless power was lost by transforming continuous variables to category variables. It has its greatest applicability in contexts in which theory is well enough developed to allow specification of the exact nature of interactive effects.

Moderated regression analysis. Cohen and Cohen (1983) have shown that any analysis of variance scheme has its analog in regression analysis. They present ANOVA models as special cases of multiple regression analysis (MRA). In the previous discussion of factorial ANOVA with correlated independent variables, we saw that a regression solution was a common way of adjusting for shared variance. MRA is a more general procedure than ANOVA which permits estimation of all types of effects, including direct, interactive, and curvilinear. When MRA is used to test interaction effects, it is referred to as moderated multiple regression (MMR) analysis. It is carried out "behind the scenes" by some ANOVA software when X and Z are correlated. MMR analysis is hierarchical, because interaction effects are always entered after the main effects of the interacting variables. The interaction effects are represented as product terms, i.e., a respondent's score on variable X is literally multiplied times his score on Z.

In most applications, MMR is used when X and Z are inherently score variables with presumed linear impacts on the criterion. The procedure should not be employed without complex adaptations when X or Z are non-linearly related to Y, when the interactive character of the variables is non-monotonic, or when X or Z have markedly skewed distributions. When assumptions are met, retaining the full score range of X and Z will normally produce a more powerful test of moderated effects than other procedures. If a variable is a natural category variable, it can be represented as a dummy variable (or variables) and the potentially interacting score variable can be multiplied by the dummy coded values.

Early suspicions regarding the serviceability of MMR analysis seem to have been effectively addressed, so they will not be discussed here (see Cohen, 1978). Attention must be given, of course, to the possible violation of regression analysis assumptions, particularly homoscedasticity, which may produce false moderators that disappear with transformation (Stone & Hollenbeck, 1989). The only important modification recently introduced in MMR is the use of "mean deviation" scores for obtaining product terms rather than the raw scores (Finney et al., 1984; Cronbach, 1987). In present practice, the means of independent variables are subtracted from respondent scores before the product term is formed. In other words, the interaction term is the product of two mean deviation scores. In earlier applications of the technique, some researchers used mean deviation or z-transformed scores to avoid the excessive collinearity of main effect and product terms that often resulted when untransformed (raw) scores were multiplied. It was thought that multicollinearity leeched power from the test of interaction terms, which may be highly redundant with previously-entered main effects.

Since MMR analysis is a special case of hierarchical MRA, the researcher should have a logical or theoretical basis for the order in which main effects are entered. The analyst should be aware that a later entered main effect is estimated after controlling for previously entered effects, so only its explanation of Y variance unshared with earlier variables is reflected. Interaction effects must be assessed after the main effects of the variables that compose them have been accounted for, since the product term reflects the confounded impact of interactive and main effects.

A test for differences between slopes as a substitute for (as opposed to a supplement to) MMR is not generally recommended (see, e.g., Jaccard et al., 1990). In the case that a bilinear interaction of an ordinal form is predicted from established theory, it may, however, be preferred to MMR. In this situation, MMR lacks power to detect a significant interaction, a problem we encountered earlier in reference to factorial ANOVA. A test for comparing slopes is available in Cohen and Cohen (1983, p. 56) and Kleinbaum and Kupper (1978, pp. 99-100). The researcher might consider trichotimizing the moderator as a hedge against unanticipated curvilinearity, though this slightly complicates the statistical testing of slope differences.

Interpretation of interactions based on comparing slopes after dichotomizing the moderator variable is, however, a limited procedure. It is geared to reflecting differences in slopes, rather than shapes, of the regression, i.e., it assumes that the interaction is of the standard "bilinear" type. Jaccard et al. (1990) recommend that interpretation be based on the metric coefficient of the product term, which indicates the number of units that the linear slope of Y on X changes for a unit change in the moderator variable. They show that by inserting values, the researcher can demonstrate the changes in the X-Y relationship as a function of the moderator.

Champoux (Champoux, 1981; Champoux & Peters, 1987) suggests examination of the regression surface to assist in interpretation of bilinear and more complex interactions. He notes that the increment in R-squared occurring with entrance of a product term in hierarchical regression is useful to reflect statistical significance, but insufficient to show the strength or size of the interaction. He recommends tabular presentation of predicted Y scores for values of the X and Z variables at the mean and one standard deviation above and below the mean. The magnitude of change in the predicted Y can be seen as a function of changes in the Z (moderator) variable. Comparisons of predicted Y values for a model including only main effects can also be presented. Champoux also proposes a standardized measure of the rate of change in the slope due to a moderator variable that can be used across studies and variables. Finally, Champoux's monte carlo research suggests that sample sizes of at least 200 are required to detect weak, but real, moderated effects, and that even larger samples are needed in the presence of considerable measurement error.

Not every technical issue regarding the use of MMR analysis is settled. There continues to be concern that the procedure lacks sufficient power to detect many real interactions (Cronbach, 1987). A more serious power problem arises when there is a large measurement error in the product term. This condition occurs when a constituent (main effect predictor) is measured with error. If one or more of the predictors used in a product term has a reliability less than .80, the interaction test may lose considerable power, especially if the sample size and effect size is low. Busemeyer and Jones (1983) and Jaccard et al. (1990) provide thorough discussions of this problem. Feucht (1989) has pointed out that attempted solutions to the problem of excessive measurement error in product terms typically assume normally distributed variables (such as LISREL), and/or multiple measurement of latent variables (such as the approach offered by Kenny & Judd, 1984). Feucht compared some estimation procedures that are based on *single* measures of each latent variable with the ordinary least squares, OLS, (uncorrected) solution. The corrected estimates, which involved adjustments of the observed moment matrices, resulted in somewhat less bias and lower standard errors than the OLS solution. It would seem that the correction procedures Feucht implemented, along with reliabilities of at least .80 and sample sizes around 100 might produce satisfactory tests for some social science research. When sample sizes are not small and reliabilities are in the 80's, Dunlap and Kemery (1987) reported little power loss, even with uncorrected OLS. Recent modifications of LISREL may also diminish the measurement error problem in tests of models with interaction terms (see Jaccard et al., 1990).

A rather different type of problem involving nonlinearity in the assessment of interaction effects with MMR was described by Veiel (1987). He shows how interactions effects, such as the classic buffering effect of social support, may arise spuriously in nomothetic research in which the outcome variable has an "off/on" quality. Depression, Veiel argues, may be regarded as a phenomenon that occurs when an individual exceeds a personal threshold of adversity. The function describing the occurrence of depression in individuals would, therefore, be a discontinuous ("step") function, rather than linear. Summing across individuals with different thresholds produces a false linearity, and ultimately an apparent bilinear interaction in MMR analysis when an additive model might be more appropriate. Veiel's analysis seems limited to outcome variables of a particular character, but raises a useful caveat where applicable.

CONCLUSIONS

This paper examined in detail the two most prevalent procedures for detecting and evaluating statistical interactions or moderated effects: factorial ANOVA and moderated regression analysis. The latter procedure (MMR) is the more general. It has undergone a number of refinements and extensions, since its origin in the middle 1950's. Whereas most applications have been in psychology, sociology, and the study of organizations, MMR analysis is a procedure that should come to have increased usage in program evaluation and other specializations in social work research. Guidelines for satisfactory research involving moderated effects parallel general recommendations for sound research: hypothesis tests should arise from clearly articulated theory, measures with high reliability and validity should be developed, and adequate sample sizes should be employed to guard against both Type I and Type II error. These standard recommendations require special emphasis because of the complex and multivariate character of research on moderated effects.

REFERENCES

Baron, R. M. & Kenny, D. A. (1986). The moderator-mediator variable distinction in social psychological research: Conceptual, strategic, and statistical considerations. *Journal of Personality and Social Psychology, 51,* 1173-1182.

Busemeyer, J. R. & Jones, L. E. (1983). Analysis of multiplicative combination rules when the causal variables are measured with error. *Psychological Bulletin, 93,* 549-562.

Champoux, J. E. (1981). The moderating effect of work context satisfactions on the curvilinear relationship between job scope and affective response. *Human Relations, 34,* 503-515.

Champoux, J. E. & Peters, W. S. (1987). Form, effect size, and power in moderated regression analysis. *Journal of Occupational Psychology, 60,* 243-255.

Cohen, J. (1978). Partialed products *are* interactions; partialed powers *are* curve components. *Psychological Bulletin, 85,* 858-866.

Cohen, J. & Cohen, P. (1983). *Applied multiple regression/correlation analysis for the behavioral sciences.* Hillsdale, New Jersey: Lawrence Erlbaum Associates.

Cook, T. D. & Campbell, D. T. (1979). *Quasi-experimentation: Design and analysis issues for field settings.* Chicago: Rand McNally.

Cooley, E. J. & Keesey, J. C. (1981). Moderator variables in life stress and illness relationship. *Journal of Human Stress, 7,* 35-40.

Cronbach, L. J. (1987). Statistical tests for moderator variables: Flaws in analyses recently proposed. *Psychological Bulletin, 102,* 414-417.

Dunlap, W. P. & Kemery, E. R. (1987). Failure to detect moderating effects: Is multicollinearity the problem? *Psychological Bulletin, 102,* 418-420.

Feucht, T. E. (1989). Estimating multiplicative regression terms in the presence of measurement error. *Sociological Methods & Research, 17,* 257-282.

Fienberg, S. E. (1977). *The analysis of cross-classified categorical data.* Cambridge: MIT Press.

Finney, J. W., Mitchell, R. E., Cronkite, R. C., & Moos, R. H. (1984). Methodological issues in estimating main and interactive effects: Examples from coping/social support and stress field. *Journal of Health and Social Behavior, 25,* 85-98.

Ghiselli, E. E. (1963). Moderating effects and differential reliability and validity. *Journal of Applied Psychology, 47,* 81-86.

Green, P. E. (1978). An AID/Logit procedure for analyzing large multiway contingency tables. *Journal of Marketing Research, 15,* 132-136.

Jaccard, J., Turrisi, R., & Wan, C. K. (1990). *Interaction effects in multiple regression.* Newbury Park, California: Sage.

Judd, C. M. & Kenny, D. A. (1981). *Estimating the effects of social interventions.* Cambridge: Cambridge University Press.

Kenny, D. A. & Judd, C. M. (1984). Estimating the nonlinear and interactive effects of latent variables. *Psychological Bulletin, 96,* 201-210.

Kleinbaum, D. G. & Kupper, L. L. (1978). *Applied regression analysis and other multivariate methods.* North Scituate, Massachusetts: Duxbury Press.

Koeske, G. F. & Koeske, R. D. (1975). Deviance and a generalized disposition toward internality: An attributional approach. *Journal of Personality, 43,* 634-646.

Koeske, G. F. & Koeske, R. D. (In Press). A preliminary test of a stress-strain-outcome model for reconceptualizing the burnout phenomenon. *Journal of Social Service Research.*

Koeske, G. F. & Koeske, R. D. (1990). Underestimation of social support buffering. Unpublished manuscript.

Koestner, R, Bernieri, F, & Zuckerman, M. (1989). Trait-specific versus person-specific moderators of cross-situational consistency. *Journal of Personality, 57,* 1-15.

Orpen, C. (1982). Type A personality as a moderator of the effects of role conflict, role ambiguity, and role overload on individual strain. *Journal of Human Stress, 8,* 8-14.

Paunonen, S. V. & Jackson, D. N. (1988). Type I error rates for moderated multiple regression analysis. *Journal of Applied Psychology, 73,* 569-573.

Rosenthal, R. & Rosnow, R. L. (1985). *Contrast analysis: Focused comparisons in the analysis of variance.* Cambridge: Cambridge University Press.

Rosenthal, R. & Rubin, D. B. (1984). Multiple contrasts and ordered Bonferroni procedures. *Psychological Bulletin, 76,* 1028-1034.

Saunders, D. R. (1956). Moderator variables in prediction. *Educational and Psychological Measurement, 16,* 209-222.

Stone, E. F. & Hollenbeck, J. R. (1989). Clarifying some controversial issues surrounding statistical procedures for detecting moderator variables: Empirical evidence and related matters. *Journal of Applied Psychology, 74,* 3-10.

Strube, M. J. & Bobko, P. (1989). Testing hypotheses about ordinal interactions: Simulations and further comments. *Journal of Applied Psychology, 74,* 247-252.

Tabachnick, B. G. & Fidell, L. S. (1983). *Using multivariate statistics.* New York: Harper & Row.

Veiel, H. O. F. (1987). Buffer effects and threshold effects: An alternative interpretation of nonlinearities in the relationship between social support, stress, and depression. *American Journal of Community Psychology, 15,* 717-740.

Wuthnow, R. (1978). *Experimentation in American religion: The new mysticisms and their implications for the churches.* Berkeley: University of California Press.

Yamatani, H. & Koeske, G. (1984). Strategies for examining racial discrimination patterns: Limits of the classical validation method. *Journal of Social Service Research, 8,* 49-60.

Zedeck, S. (1971). Problems with the use of "moderator" variables. *Psychological Bulletin, 76,* 295-310.

Interaction Effects in Multiple Regression

Claudia Coulton
Julian Chow

SUMMARY. Multiple regression is widely used for the analysis of nonexperimental data by investigators in social work and social welfare. Most published studies test additive models in which the effects of each independent variable on the dependent variable are assumed to be constant across all levels of additional independent variables. Tests are seldom made for the presence of interaction or modifier effects. This article discusses the concept of interaction, the use of product terms to test for its presence, the problems of multicollinearity and nonlinear interaction effects and the proper use of subgroup analysis.

The concept of statistical interaction is widely understood and applied within the context of experimental design. The analysis of variance models associated with experimental data typically include a test for the presence of interaction effects. Less common are tests for interaction effects in multiple regression analyses with nonexperimental designs. In fact, a review of four social welfare

---

Claudia Coulton is Professor and Director, Center for Urban Poverty and Social Change, Mandel School of Applied Social Sciences, Case Western Reserve University, Cleveland, OH. She earned her PhD in Social Welfare at Case Western Reserve University. Her current research interests are urban poverty and the impact of neighborhood environment and economic deprivation on health status.

Julian Chow earned his MSSA and is a PhD candidate at the Mandel School of Applied Social Sciences, Case Western Reserve University. He is Research Associate and Data Manager at the Center for Urban Poverty and Social Change at the Mandel School. His major research interest is the dynamic structural change of urban neighborhoods.

Requests for reprints should be sent to Claudia Coulton, Center for Urban Poverty and Social Change, Mandel School of Applied Social Sciences, Case Western Reserve University, Cleveland, OH 44128.

© 1992 by The Haworth Press, Inc. All rights reserved.

journals (*Social Work, Social Service Review, Social Work Research and Abstracts*, and *Journal of Social Service Research*) for 1988 and 1989 revealed only two instances of ordinary least squares regression models that explicitly tested for interaction effects. Yet, theories related to social work and social welfare often contain implicit notions of interaction. The infrequency of these models suggests that researchers doing nonexperimental research may be insufficiently familiar with alternative methods of modeling these effects and issues that arise in applying these techniques.

This article covers the steps that an investigator takes in considering the possibility of interaction and modeling it statistically. The focus is on data that are nonexperimental and variables that are continuous, not categorical. It begins by describing some theoretical propositions or research questions that imply the possibility of statistical interaction. Second, it reviews the concept of interaction as generally examined in analysis of variance models. Third, it describes the standard approach to testing for interaction effects within multiple regression models. Fourth, it identifies two limitations of these standard approaches, multicollinearity and nonlinear interaction, and discusses some methods of addressing these issues. Finally, it reviews subgroup analysis that has often been used as a method of identifying interaction and discusses the limitations and appropriate use of this technique.

THEORY AND STATISTICAL INTERACTION

Propositions implying that the effects of an independent variable on a dependent variable depend upon the values of one or more other variables call for the testing of statistical interaction. Interaction effects are often referred to as conditional, and one of the variables may be referred to as a moderator variable because it modifies the relationship between an independent and dependent variable. This term ought not to be confused with a mediating variable. A mediating variable is one that comes between an independent and dependent variable in a causal chain and carries the indirect effects.

Theory may suggest several forms of interaction effects. One possibility is that of buffering. Theories regarding stress and coping often include the proposition that social support mitigates the negative effects of stress on health (Finney et al, 1984). In other words, as social support increases, the strength of the effect of stress on health is lowered. At the highest levels of support, stress would be expected to have little effect on health. Theory suggests that social support prevents the negative impact of stress because it is a coping resource, allowing the supported individual to adapt to or minimize the stress. It is seldom suggested that stress has a positive effect on health even when support is at the maximum. Its role is only to moderate negative effects and, therefore, the interaction is thought to be ordinal rather than disordinal.

A second prospect is a moderator variable that intensifies the effect of the independent variable on a dependent variable. An example of this comes from the decision making and locus of control literature (Coulton et al., 1989). Theory suggests that an individual's lack of control over a specific decision will affect the level of subsequent depression, but that the nature of this effect depends upon the individual's locus of control or expectancy. There are two possibilities for the exact form of this effect. One is a threshold effect in which there is no effect of decision making on depression until a particular threshold of locus of control is reached. The impact of decision making on depression then rises gradually above this threshold. Another possibility is a disordinal interaction: persons with an internal locus of control become more depressed as decision control declines and persons with an external locus of control become more depressed when decision control increases.

An additional type of theoretical proposition that implies statistical interaction is one that specifies a contingency or congruence effect. Person-environment fit exemplifies this type of effect (Kulka, 1979). A matching of environmental resources with personal needs of residents is anticipated to result in better outcomes while environments with too many or too few resources produce a negative outcome (Coulton, 1979; Coulton et al., 1984). In this case, the relationship between the amount of an environmental resource and outcome will be positive for those with a high need, negative for those with a low need, and curvilinear for those with a moderate need. To illustrate, consider the degree to which an environment provides opportunities for autonomy. Residents with high autonomy needs would improve as environmental autonomy rises. Those who needed little autonomy would decompensate under high autonomy conditions. Those with moderate needs would have poorer outcomes in both higher and lower autonomy environments.

The three theories described here imply distinct forms of interaction that are represented in Figure 1. The stress buffering theory is shown in Figure 1a. At high levels of support there is no relationship between stress and health. The effect of stress on health is greatest for those with little or no support. Figure 1b displays the hypothesized interaction effect when locus of control at either extreme intensifies in opposing directions the impact of decision control on depression. Figure 1c represents a person-environment fit perspective on the degree of autonomy allowed in an environment. For persons with high autonomy needs, the greater the autonomy allowed, the better their functioning. The situation is reversed for persons with low tolerance for autonomy. For persons in the middle on autonomy, the relationship between environmental autonomy and functioning is curvilinear.

The investigators first step in planning to test for statistical interaction is to determine the form of the interaction effect suggested by theory. Some theories are strong and can predict the exact shape *a priori*; others are weaker and require a more exploratory approach. Nonetheless, it is essential that the investigator

FIGURE 1. Shape of Interaction Effects

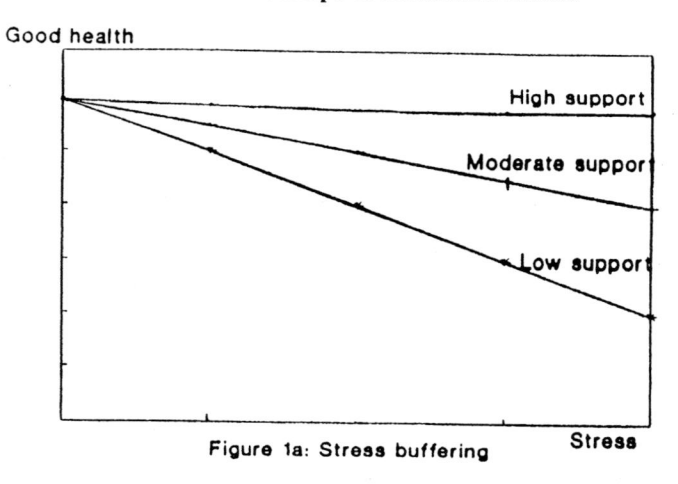

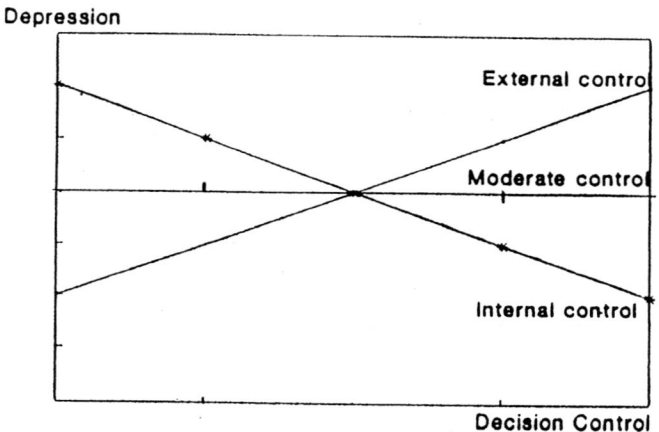

Figure 1a: Stress buffering

Figure 1b: Locus of control, intensification

Functioning

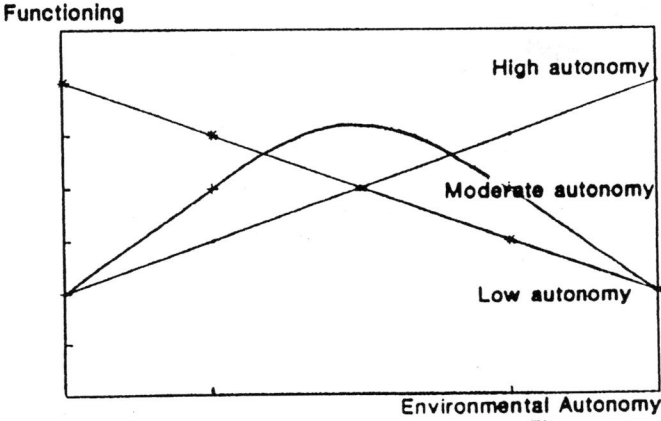

Figure 1c: Person - Environment Fit

carry out the statistical modeling of interaction with an understanding of the theoretical implications.

A BRIEF REVIEW OF INTERACTION IN ANOVA

Many researchers were first introduced to the concept of statistical interaction within the context of balanced factorial designs. The model underlying the usual analysis of variance is non-additive and includes both main and interaction effects. For two factors, A and B:

$$Y_{ijk} = \mu + \alpha_j + \beta_k + \alpha\beta_{jk} + \varepsilon_{ijk}$$

where Y_{ijk} is the score of any case on the dependent variable, μ is the grand mean, α_j is the effect of the jth level of A, β_k is the effect of the kth level of B, $\alpha\beta_{jk}$ is the interaction effect and ε_{ijk} is error.

In a two way factorial analysis of variance, the interaction hypothesis reflects differences among "twice corrected" cell means (Kennedy and Bush, 1985). The interaction sum of squares reflects the differences among cell means after the effects of A and B have been taken into account.

There are several important differences between the balanced factorial design and the nonexperimental design that are pertinent to modeling interaction effects. First, the independent variables that are hypothesized to interact are seldom orthogonal in nonexperimental research. In factorial designs, there can be no correlation between the independent variables when the cell n's are equal or proportional. The intercorrelated nature of the independent variables in much nonexperimental research can pose difficulties in interpreting the main and interaction effects. These will be discussed later in this article.

A second difference is that the ANOVA factors are categorical with no assumptions about the ordering of the levels of the factors or the shape of the interaction effects. Continuous variables in multiple regression are assumed to represent an interval scale. When modeling the interaction effects of continuous variables, it is necessary to consider the possibility that the interaction effect is not constant across all levels of the independent variables. As will be demonstrated later in this article, the model tested will need to be adjusted accordingly.

A final difference is the methods that are used to interpret interaction effects when they are uncovered. An examination of cell means and simple effects usually reveals the substantive differences responsible for interaction in ANOVA. The substantive interpretation of interaction effects following multiple regression is more complex and usually involves examining how the effect of an independent variable on a dependent variable changes over levels of a third variable. Unlike experimental designs in which an equal (or adequate) number of subjects is assigned to each level of the independent variable, nonexperimental studies reflect the distribution of the sample on the independent variables. The number of cases may be too few to perform a reliable description across all levels of the independent variable.

Interaction in Multiple Regression

The model typically tested with multiple regression is linear and additive:

$$Y = b_0 + b_1 X_1 + b_2 X_2 + e$$

Y is the dependent variable, X_1 and X_2 are independent variables, b's are regression coefficients and e is error. This model assumes that the effects of each independent variable are the same across all values of the other independent variable. In other words, interaction effects are not included. If interaction effects indeed exist, the additive model is said to be misspecified and the coefficients are biased.

It is widely accepted that interaction effects can be represented in a linear model by the inclusion of an additional term that is the product of the relevant independent variables (Allison, 1977; Cohen, 1978; Cohen & Cohen, 1983; Jaccard et al., 1990). The general form of the model is:

$$Y' = b_0 + b_1 X_1 + b_2 X_2 + b_3 X_1 X_2$$

The significance of the interaction effect can be determined using an F test that is analogous to the F for interaction in analysis of variance. It is based on the difference between the R^2 for the model that includes the interaction and the R^2 for the additive model that includes only the main effects. Because the variance accounted for by the main effects is subtracted from the variance accounted for by the model including interaction, the F test reflects the partial or pure effects of the interaction. This is analogous to the differences between "twice corrected" cell means in the ANOVA model. The formula for the F test for the R^2 increment is:

$$F = \frac{R_2^2 - R_1^2 / K_2 - K_1}{1 - R_2^2 / N - K_2 - 1}$$

R_2^2 is the R^2 for the model that includes the interaction term. R_1^2 is the R^2 for the model that includes only main effects. K_2 and K_1 are the respective number of independent variables in the model.

An Example

A set of data will be used to illustrate these steps and the points made later in this article. While the substance of the example is drawn from the authors' actual research, the data have been modified to exemplify some important difficulties and issues that often arise in modeling interaction effects.

Consider a study of elderly patients in an acute care hospital who are making decisions about their post-hospital care. The literature suggests that many patients suffer dissatisfaction and reactive depression upon relocating from the hospital to an ongoing care setting. Some studies indicate that depression is greatest among persons who lack control over the decision. Yet other studies find patients lacking in control who are not depressed. This mix of findings is consistent with the possibility that the effect of decision control on depression or dissatisfaction may depend on a third factor. In this study, the investigators hypothesize that the patient's locus of control will determine or modify the effect of decision control on an outcome such as depression. In other words, an interaction effect is expected.

It is important prior to beginning their analysis that the investigators consider the nature of this interaction effect. In this case, they are confident that persons with a highly internal locus of control will experience a strong inverse effect of decision control on depression, i.e., the higher the decision control, the lower the depression. For those with an external locus of control they believe two outcomes are possible: (1) there will be no relationship between decision control and depression; or (2) there will be a positive effect with higher control leading to more depression. Although in reality the investigators also include additional independent and control variables, these will be omitted from this example to focus on the modeling and interpretation of interaction effects.

The four variables for this analysis are described in Table 1. High scores are indicative of greater depression and decision control and a more internal locus of control. The reader should note that the interaction variable (i.e., the product

Table 1: Descriptive Statistics for Example

	Mean	Std. Dev.	Y_1	Correlation X_1	X_2	$(X_1 * X_2)$
Depression (Y_1)	53.73	17.25				
Decision-making Control (X_1)	5.29	1.66	-.391			
Internal LOC (X_2)	5.57	2.84	.193	-.281		
Raw Interaction ($X_1 * X_2$)	28.14	15.63	-.281	.409	.714	
Centered Interaction $(X_1-\bar{X_1})*(X_2-\bar{X_2})$	-1.31	4.89	-.752	.279	-.258	.230

term) is substantially correlated with the independent variables. This multicollinearity will cause some difficulties that will be discussed later.

The results of the regression analysis of the non-additive model are presented in Table 2. The variables have been entered into the model in order of main effects first followed by the interaction effects. The regression coefficients that are presented, however, are based on the full model.

The first step is to examine the F value for the R^2 increment for the interaction term. In this case it is significant, suggesting the presence of an interaction effect. The slope or unstandardized regression coefficient (b) for the interaction variable can be interpreted as the amount of change in the slope of depression on decision control that is estimated for a unit change in locus of control. The b of -2.49 for interaction suggests that as locus of control goes up, the slope of control on depression goes down or becomes more negative.

The interpretation of regression coefficients for the main effects is not straight forward, and some have suggested that they not be interpreted at all (Smith and Sasaki, 1979). Nevertheless, the main effects can be interpreted if it is noted that they now represent conditional effects rather than the overall effects that are obtained in an additive model. The main effects' coefficients are the slopes of Y on X when the other X variable is zero. In this example, the coefficient for decision control suggests that depression increases by 11.73 for each unit of increase in control for persons whose locus of control is zero. The difficulty in using this finding is that locus of control is not measured on a ratio scale and a value of zero has no apparent meaning. The next section will discuss a transformation that can aid interpretation of main effects.

The Problem of Multicollinearity

As noted earlier, the interaction term in this model is highly correlated with the independent variables that were used to form the product variable. This multicollinearity can often be extreme, especially when the independent variables are themselves intercorrelated. Multicollinearity in multiple regression produces problems in calculating the regression coefficients and increases their standard errors. When multicollinearity is extreme, one or more variables are almost perfect linear combinations of other variables in the matrix. Under these circumstances, necessary matrix manipulations cannot take place or result in considerable error.

That multicollinearity is present in the example used here can be seen in several ways. First, the standardized regression coefficients (Betas) exceed one as a result of calculation errors. Second, the tolerance for all of the variables is low, less than .1 for two of the three variables. The tolerance represents the variance in each variable that is not explained by other variables in the matrix. A low tolerance is evidence that one variable has extreme multicollinearity with other variables.

Table 2: Raw Score Regression Analysis Example[1]

	b	Beta	Tolerance
DM Control (X_1)	11.74**(1.99)	1.13**(.19)	.153
LOC (X_2)	12.89**(1.52)	2.12**(.25)	.096
R^2=.1607*			
Interaction ($X_1 * X_2$)	-2.49**(.29)	-2.26**(.26)	.087
R^2 change = .4427* (F=73.66)			

----
*p<.05
**p<.001

[1]Standard errors are given in parentheses. The regression coefficients are for the full model, with both main and interaction effects included.

Centering has been suggested as a method of reducing multicollinearity in regression models with interaction terms (Cronbach, 1987; Smith & Sasaki, 1979; Tate, 1984). The independent variables are transformed into deviation scores by subtracting the mean from each score. The deviation scores are then used to create the product term. Thus, the regression model tested is:

$$Y' = b_0 + b_1(X_1 - \overline{X}_1) + b_2(X_2 - \overline{X}_2) + b_3[(X_1 - \overline{X}_1)(X_2 - \overline{X}_2)]$$

The use of deviation scores results in two benefits: multicollinearity is reduced and the regression coefficients for the main effects become easier to interpret. The effects of centering on multicollinearity can be seen in Table 3, where the previous example is now tested using deviation scores. The Betas are now less than one as they should be and the standard errors for the regression coefficients are lower. The tolerances for all variables are within an acceptable range.

Using centered scores has not changed the R^2 increment for interaction nor the F value. The unstandardized regression coefficient for the interaction term is also the same as it was in the raw score equation.

The regression coefficients for the main effects have changed and now require a different, and more useful, interpretation than the coefficients for the raw scores. The coefficients now can be interpreted as the slope of the dependent variable on the independent variable when the other independent variable is at its mean. For example, the slope of depression on decision control is -2.16 for individuals who score at the mean on locus of control.

The investigator will be aided in understanding the substantive implications of the interaction coefficient by calculating the predicted slope for subjects with selected values of locus of control (see Figure 1). The equation for these calculations is:

$$b_1 \text{ at } X_2 = b_1 + b_3 X_2$$

For persons with locus of control scores of 2 (very external) and 9 (very internal) respectively, we can substitute their *deviation* scores in the above equation and predict the following slopes. For locus of control equal to 2 (i.e., deviation score of -3.57):

$$b_1 \text{ at } X_2 = -2.16 + [(-2.49)(-3.57)] = 6.72$$

For locus of control equal to 9 (i.e., deviation score of 3.43):

$$b_1 \text{ at } X_2 = -2.16 + [(-2.49)(3.43)] = -10.70$$

Table 3: Centered Score Regression Analysis Example[1]

	b	Beta	Tolerance
DM Control (x_1)	-2.16*(.86)	-.21*(.08)	.875
LOC (x_2)	-.29 (.49)	-.05 (.08)	.886
R^2=.1607*			
Interaction ($x_1 * x_2$)	-2.49**(.29)	-.71**(.08)	.837
R^2 change = .4427** (F=73.66)			

----

*p<.05
**p<.001

[1]Standard errors are given in parentheses. The regression coefficients are for the full model, with both main and interaction effects included.

190

The model predicts a moderate positive effect of decision control on depression for the extreme external and a strongly negative effect for the extreme internals. The estimated intercept for the X_2 group is equal to $b_2 X_2 + a$.

The Form of the Interaction Effect

The product term, either raw or centered, represents a particular form of interaction, one that is bilinear. In other words, it correctly models the situation where the change in the slope of the dependent variable on the independent variable is monotonic and uniform across all levels of the third variable.

Some theoretical propositions explicitly depart from this assumption. If, for example, the slope of Y on X_1 is expected to be high at the mean of X_2 but low when scores on X_2 are at either extreme, the predicted form of the interaction effect would be quadratic, not linear. A study in which the number of counseling sessions affects symptom reduction for people who have levels of disability in the middle range but has less impact on symptom reduction among people with very mild or severe disabilities is an illustration of this type of interaction effect.

Prior to conducting the analysis, the investigator may not be sure about the form of the interaction effect but cannot assume monotonicity and uniformity. As an exploratory technique, slopes of Y on X_1 can be calculated using subsamples with scores in selected ranges of X_2 to see whether the amount and direction of the change in slopes is constant or varies. This will help the investigator to substantively interpret the interaction effect and also decide whether to include a squared or higher order term in the model to represent a nonlinear component of the interaction. However, because small subsample sizes may make these estimates unreliable, these should be interpreted cautiously.

To illustrate, the slopes of depression on decision control are calculated for subjects at four levels of locus of control. For the group with locus of control scores of less than 3 (extreme externals) the slope is 12.13 indicating that more decision control leads to greater depression in this subgroup. For moderate externals (locus of control scores from 3 through 5), the slope is 4.73 and not significant. For modest internals (locus of control scores from 6 through 8), the slope is -7.08. And for extreme internals (locus of control scores greater than 8), the slope is -9.42, indicating that lower decision control is associated with more depression (see Figure 2).

An examination of these slopes suggests that the change goes from a high value (12.13) to a low value (-9.42) as locus of control increases. In other words, the trend is continuously decreasing or monotonic as it moves along the points of the locus of control scale. However, the rate of decrease is not constant; it is greater at the external end than at the internal end of the scale. It is, therefore, possible that there is a quadratic component to the interaction effect.

A quadratic interaction effect can be tested in the same way that linear and quadratic effects can be tested in multiple regression; through the inclusion of a squared term in a polynomial (Cohen & Cohen, 1983). The form of the model is:

FIGURE 2. Linear Effects

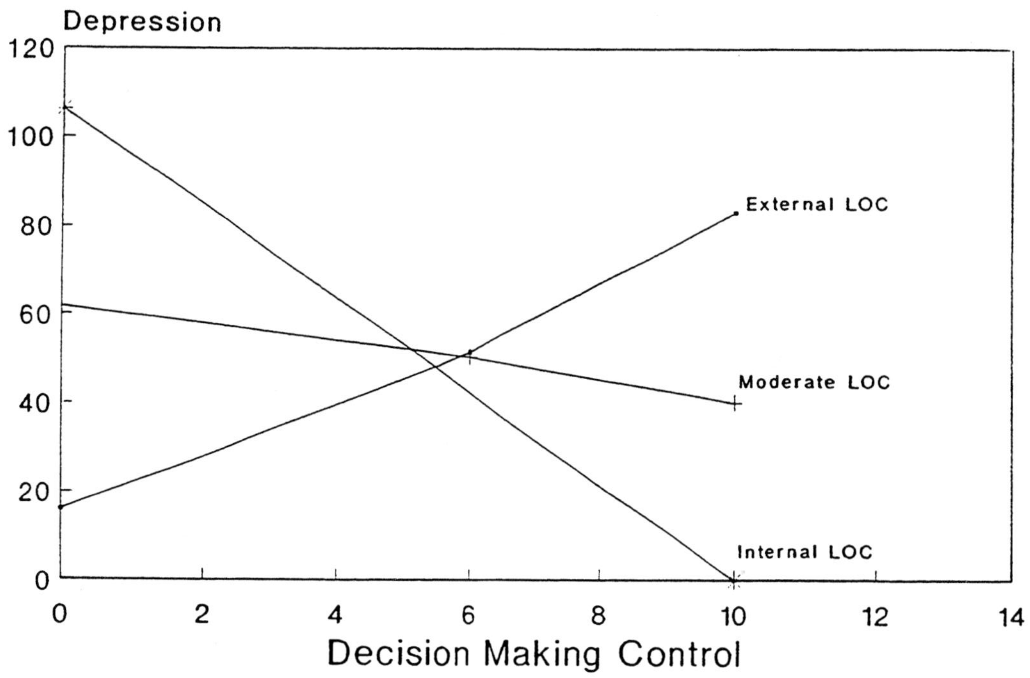

$$Y' = b_0 + b_1 X_1 + b_2 X_2 + b_3 X_2^2 + b_4 X_1 X_2 + b_5 X_1 X_2^2$$

The R^2 increment for both the linear and squared interaction term represents the entire interaction effect in this case.

The possibility of a quadratic interaction effect is tested in Table 4 in which the centered product term is entered along with the product of X_1 and X_2 squared. It can be seen that the R^2 increment for the squared term is significant. The interaction effect is represented more accurately by the combined R^2 increment for both the product term and the squared product term.

Figure 3 displays the interaction effect including the nonlinear component. The quadratic model more accurately represents that the change in the slope of depression on decision making is greatest at the external end of the locus of control continuum. Interaction effects may take many other nonlinear forms. The investigator may need to consider logarithmic transformations, square root transformation or other methods of more closely representing the actual shape of the interaction effect.

Threshold Effects

One additional type of interaction, a threshold effect, may require the addition of dummy variables to a model. A threshold effect is one in which X_1 has little or no effect on Y until some threshold is reached on X_2. Above the threshold, the effect increases rapidly. Recent thinking about the effects of concentrated poverty on neighborhood decline imply threshold effects (Coulton et al., 1990). Population turnover and crime rates are only weakly related for neighborhoods below 40% or 50% poverty rates. Above the threshold, the slope increases rapidly.

This type of effect can be modeled by including a dummy (0,1) variable indicating whether a neighborhood is above or below the threshold. If the theory is correct, the investigator would see that the slope of crime on population turnover is relatively flat and unchanged for poverty rates at points along the continuum from 0% to 40%. Then the slope shifts markedly as the rate rises from 40% to 100%. Under these circumstances, the interaction effect would be better represented by including both a linear product term as well as a product term with the dummy variable.

Using Subgroup Analysis

It is not uncommon for researchers to address the possibility of moderator or interaction effects indirectly through the use of subgroup analysis. Rather than including the moderator variable as a product term in a regression analysis, the sample is split at the median or some other point on the moderator variable. Separate regression analyses are performed and compared.

This technique has several limitations when it is used as the primary method of detecting interaction. First, information is lost when a continuous variable is split. The assumption is made that the effect of the independent variable on the

Table 4: Non-linear Regression Analysis Example[1]

	b	Beta	Tolerance
DM Control (x_1)	-5.22**(1.34)	-.50**(.13)	.330
LOC (x_2)	-.17 (.48)	-.03 (.08)	.871
R^2=.1607*			
x_2^2	.04(.25)	.02(.09)	.709
R^2 change = .0002 (F=.0148)			

$x_1 * x_2$	$-2.65^{**}(.28)$	$-.75^{**}(.08)$	.855
	R^2 change $= .4489^{**}(F=74.76)$		
$x_1 * x_2^2$	$.36^{*}(.13)$	$.39^{*}(.14)$	.264
	R^2 change $= .0405^{*}(F=7.40)$		

---

*p<.05
**p<.001

[1]Standard errors are given in parentheses. The regression coefficients are for the full model, with both main and interaction effects included.

FIGURE 3. Quadratic Effects

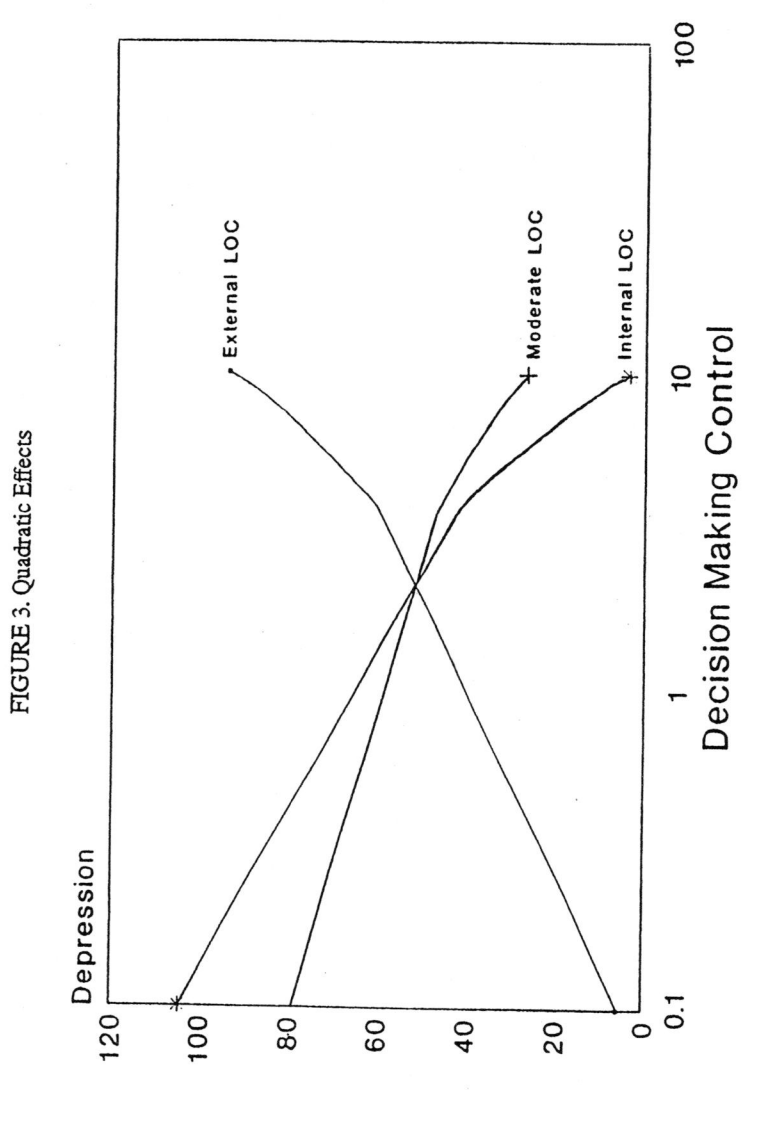

dependent variable is constant across the multiple levels of the moderator variable represented in the subgroup. Further, the cut-points that are chosen can affect the results and conclusions may differ based on where they are drawn (Cronbach and Snow, 1977).

A second flaw in many examples of subgroup analysis is that multiple correlation coefficients rather than slopes are compared. Under these circumstances, interaction effects cannot be distinguished from homologizer effects (Sharma et al., 1981). It is possible that a grouping variable results in one sample having a smaller error term than another because the grouping variable is correlated with error (Zedeck, 1971). The R^2 is larger because the error variance is smaller, not because the relationship between the independent and dependent variable is stronger.

For example, suppose that recent adult immigrants were found to have a weaker correlation between their arthritis pain scores and their visits to the physician than were persons who immigrated as children. A researcher could mistakenly conclude that recent immigrants were less inclined to use medical care in response to pain than early immigrants when the real difference between the samples is in the error variance. Greater error variance could be due to the measurement of pain being less reliable in the recent immigrant group or to the fact that this group has important determinants of individual differences in use of medical care that are omitted from the model.

The misleading effects of differences in error variances across subgroups can be eliminated by comparing unstandardized regression coefficients rather than multiple correlation coefficients. If there are valid reasons to believe that there is homogeneity of slopes within subgroups and heterogeneity across subgroups, then the cut-points used to establish these groups may have theoretical justification. Under these circumstances, pairs of unstandardized regression coefficients can be tested for the significance of their differences (Cohen and Cohen, 1983:56).

However, when more than one subgroup is involved, it is preferable to code the subgroups as k-1 dummy variables and to form product terms between this set of coded variables and the independent variable for inclusion in the regression analysis. The overall interaction effect is represented by the R^2 increment for the group of product terms. The focus on the significance of the R^2 increment holds the overall probability of a type two error at the designated alpha. Multiple, pairwise comparisons among regression coefficients inflate the actual alpha beyond the designated level.

CONCLUSIONS

Investigators doing nonexperimental research related to social welfare and social work need to give greater consideration to models that include statistical interaction. They should explicitly link theory to the statistical model to be used, rather than automatically assuming an additive model. Social work and social welfare researchers may be insufficiently aware of the fact that leaving out a valid interaction effect causes their models to be misspecified. The coefficients that are obtained in such a model could be misleading because they are constrained to be equal at all levels of the independent variable.

Being precise about the form that interaction may take is particularly important, since it often departs from the bilinear model represented by simple product term analysis. Exploration of differences in slopes among subgroups may be helpful in understanding the form of the effect when the investigator does not have an *a priori* hypothesis. However, these subgroup slopes must be interpreted with caution due to decreased sample size. They may generally be taken as suggestive of alternative forms of models that are then tested within the context of the multiple regression equation.

The comparison of correlation coefficients across subgroups formed by making a continuous variable into a categorical one is to be discouraged in most circumstances, because these correlation coefficients can be affected by differences in error variances and restriction of range. Unstandardized regression coefficients can be compared across subgroups, but the cut-points for subgroup formation should have some basis in theory.

REFERENCES

Allison, P. H. (1977). Testing for interaction in multiple regression. *American Journal of Sociology, 83*, 144-153.

Cohen, J. (1978). Partialed products are interactions; partialed powers are curve components. *Psychological Bulletin, 85*, 858-866.

Cohen, J., & Cohen, P. (1983). *Applied multiple regression for the behavioral sciences* (2nd ed.). Hillsdale NJ: Lawrence Earlbaum.

Coulton, C. J. (1979). Developing an instrument to measure person-environment fit. *Journal of Social Service Research, 3*(2), 159-174.

Coulton, C. J., Dunkle, R. E., Haug, M., Chow, J., & Vielhaber, D. P. (1989). Locus of control and decision making for posthospital care. *The Gerontologist, 29*(5), 627-632.

Coulton, C. J., Holland, T., & Fitch, V. (1984). Person-environment congruence and psychiatric patient outcome in community care homes. *Administration in Mental Health, 12*, 71-88.

Coulton, C. J., Pandey, S., & Chow J. (1990). Concentration of poverty and the changing ecology of low-income, urban neighborhoods. *Social Work Research and Abstracts, 26* (4).

Cronbach, L. J. (1987). Statistical tests for moderator variables: Flaws in analyses recently proposed. *Psychological Bulletin, 102*, 414-417.

Cronbach, L. J., & Snow, R. E. (1977). *Aptitudes and instructional methods: A handbook for research on interactions.* New York: Irvington.

Finney, J. W., Mitchell, R. E., Cronkite, R. C., & Moos, R. H. (1984). Methodological issues in estimating main and interactive effects: Examples from coping/social support and stress field. *Journal of Health and Social Behavior, 25,* 85-98.

Jaccard, J., Turrisi, R., & Wan, C. K. (1990). *Interaction effects in multiple regression,* Newbury Park, CA: Sage.

Kennedy, J. J., & Bush, A. J. (1985). *An introduction to the design and analysis of experiments in behavioral research,* Lanham, MD: University Press of America.

Kulka, R. A. (1979). Interaction as person-environment fit. In L. R. Kahle (ed.), *Methods for studying person-situation interactions* (pp. 55-72). San Francisco: Jossey-Bass.

Sharma, S., Durand, R. M., & Gur-Arie, O. (1981). Identification and analysis of moderator variables. *Journal of Marketing Research, 18,* 291-300.

Smith, W., & Sasaki, M. S. (1979). Decreasing multicollinearity: A method for models with multiplicative functions. *Sociological Methods and Research 8,* 35-56.

Tate, R. L. (1984). Limitations of centering for interactive models. *Sociological Methods and Research, 13,* 251-271.

Zedeck, S. (1971). Problems with the use of moderator variables. *Psychological Bulletin, 76,* 295-310.

Social Network Analysis

Calvin L. Streeter
David F. Gillespie

SUMMARY. Network analysis is presented as a useful extension of conventional forms of analysis. We introduce and illustrate basic features of network analysis. Reference materials are suggested and data from a network of 80 emergency service organizations are used to illustrate a matrix approach to network analysis. Our discussion shows how network analysis can complement standard modes of analysis to broaden and deepen the application of theories to social work. We conclude that network analysis has great potential in social work research and theory.

Network analysis is becoming increasingly popular as a general methodology for understanding complex patterns of interaction. The network perspective

---

Calvin L. Streeter received his PhD from the George Warren Brown School of Social Work at Washington University in St. Louis. He is currently Assistant Professor in the School of Social Work at the University of Texas at Austin. He continues to do research in the area of disaster planning and preparedness, and is currently developing a clinical assessment instrument to examine social support among adolescents. He is also involved in a feasibility study of the Food Stamp Employment and Training Program for the Texas Department of Human Services.

David F. Gillespie is Professor, George Warren Brown School of Social Work, Washington University, St. Louis, MO 63130.

Collection of the data for this work was supported by the National Science Foundation (NSF), Societal Response to Earthquake Hazards Mitigation Program, Grant No. CEE-8314421. The analyses and writing were accomplished with support from the National Science Foundation, Grant No. BCS-8920472. Any opinions, findings, conclusions, or recommendations expressed in this publication are those of the authors and do not necessarily reflect the views of the National Science Foundation.

The authors express their appreciation to Charles Glisson, University of Tennessee, and Susan A. Murty, Washington University, for comments and suggestions which improved the paper.

Requests for reprints should be sent to Calvin L. Streeter, School of Social Work, The University of Texas at Austin, Austin, TX 78712.

© 1992 by The Haworth Press, Inc. All rights reserved.

examines actors which are connected directly or indirectly by one or more different relationships. Any theoretically meaningful unit of analysis may be treated as actors: individuals, groups, organizations, communities, states, or countries. Regardless of unit level, network analysis describes structure and patterns of relationships, and seeks to understand both their causes and consequences.

While the network concept has deep roots in anthropology and sociology (Bott, 1955; Moreno, 1934), standard techniques for studying the structure of social networks have been a relatively recent development. Several factors contribute to the growing popularity of network analysis in the social sciences. For one thing, the world is becoming more interdependent as reflected in overlapping corporate boards, international markets, specialized service economies, and the involvement of multiple levels of government in many aspects of daily life. Another factor is the applicability of network analysis across different units and levels of analysis. As Burt (1980) points out, network analysis is a potentially powerful methodology for connecting micro and macro levels of social theory. A third factor has been advances in computer technology which make it possible to design network studies and conduct complex network analyses which were impossible just a decade ago.

The purpose of this paper is to encourage wider use of network analysis in social work. We do this by introducing and illustrating basic features of network analysis, and by presenting a network analysis of an interorganizational network. This analysis is performed using a software package called STRUCTURE, Version 4.1 (Burt, 1989). This software was selected because it provides the most advanced package now available for the personal computer. Like most network analysis packages, it produces basic network measures such as density, centrality, and structural equivalence, and it is relatively easy to use because of a new "ASSISTANT" module which helps generate the command statements needed to conduct the analysis. In addition, STRUCTURE contains procedures for testing the reliability of measures and testing hypotheses related to network structures. Our discussion also shows how network analysis can be incorporated with conventional forms of analysis to broaden and deepen the theoretical questions raised in social work.

PROPERTIES OF SOCIAL NETWORKS

A social network can be defined as any bounded set of connected social units. This definition highlights three important characteristics of social networks. First, networks have boundaries. That is, some criterion exists to determine membership in the network. In some networks, such as family systems, friendship groups, and work teams, boundaries are relatively straight-forward and easy to define. But social networks are also presumed to be embedded in larger social systems. Therefore, it is sometimes difficult to distinguish between a network and its broader social context. The definition of boundaries is a critical first step toward the study of social networks.

The second key element of the definition is "connectedness" in social networks. To be part of a social network, each member must have either actual or potential links to at least one other member of the network. These links may be direct or indirect. While some members may be peripheral in the network or almost completely isolated, each one must somehow be connected to other members if it is to be considered part of the network.

The third key aspect of this definition is the social unit. Network analysis can be easily applied to a wide range of social units. They can be individuals, as in the case of social support networks. But they can also be social service agencies, social institutions in local communities, or nations in the global economy. In a diverse profession like social work, social network analysis has direct applications for the study of clinical practice, social policy analysis, community organization, and organizational management.

The concept of social network embodies a complex set of social phenomena and studies of social networks have examined a diverse set of properties. As a way of summarizing these properties, we have classified them into two major categories: relational properties and structural properties. Table 1 presents a brief summary of the properties under these two dimensions.

Relational properties focus on the content of the relationship between network members and on the form of these relationships. Studies of relational properties typically seek to understand why a network exists and to ascertain the functions performed by the relations among the members. Two aspects of relational properties have been studied: transaction content, and the nature of relationships. Transaction content refers to what flows or what is exchanged in networks. Four basic types of exchange content have been identified: resources, information, influence, and social support. The nature of relationships refers to the qualities inherent in the relationship between members of the network.

While relational properties deal with the content of relations, structural properties describe the way members fit together to form social networks. Structural characteristics of networks can be divided into three levels of analysis: individual members, sub-groups, and total networks. Measures of individual members describe differences among their connections to other members of the network. These differences can be used to identify individual roles in the network, such as star, liaison, bridge, and gatekeeper (Tichy and Fombrun, 1979; Paulson, 1985). Measures with subgroups as the unit of analysis represent the structural characteristics of clusters within the total network. Most social networks contain areas of concentration which have more linkages or connections between members than others. These concentrations are examined as clusters. Measures used at this level describe both the structural characteristics of the sub-group itself, and how the subgroup fits into the total network. When

Table 1

Properties of Social Networks

Relational properties

    Transaction content
        Resources: physical goods, personnel, services
        Information: descriptions, opinions, ideas, facts
        Influence: power, prestige, legitimation, advice
        Social support: comfort, encouragement, inspiration

    Nature of the relationship
        Importance: significance of the relationship
        Frequency: rate of recurrence
        Formalization: official recognition
        Standardization: defined procedures and units of exchange

Structural properties

    Individual members of the network
        Centrality: number of linkages relative to other members
        Connectedness: membership in more than one sub-group
        Distance: number of links connecting two members

    Subgroups
        Number: Number of subgroups
        Size: Number of members in each subgroup
        Connectedness: extent to which sub-groups are connected
        Openness: number of linkages out from the sub-group

    Total network
        Size: number of members in the network
        Density: ratio of actual to potential connections
        Hierarchy: extent to which connections are directed upward
        Centrality: degree to which connections are directed
            through one or a few central units in the network

the total network is the unit of analysis, it is not partitioned into subgroups. The measures used at this level describe the overall patterns of relationship among all members of the network.

APPROACHES TO NETWORK ANALYSIS

The term network analysis refers to a loose federation of approaches (Burt, 1980). While these approaches are all designed to increase our understanding of the network as a system, they vary greatly in complexity and focus. Several authors have provided excellent reviews of various approaches to network analysis (Burt, 1980; 1982; Knoke and Kuklinski, 1982; Paulson, 1985; DiMaggio, 1986). These reviews are quite technical, presenting a variety of approaches for describing and analyzing network data.[1] Our approach introduces the basic concepts necessary to begin using network analysis. We discuss two approaches to network analysis: graph models and matrix models.

Graph Models

Visual imagery has played a significant role in network analysis since its inception. Drawing on the pioneering work of Moreno (1934), most graphic models of networks are presented as sociograms which display the relations among network members in two dimensional space. Members of the network are represented as points or nodes, with lines drawn between pairs of nodes to show a relationship between them. An arrow is sometimes used to show the direction of flow in a relationship.

There are several practical advantages to using graphic models. Graphic displays of relations between network members can convey a vivid image of the network. They can also produce an intuitive understanding of structure which is difficult to achieve any other way. In fact, some have argued that points and lines are the most "natural" way to represent social networks (Klovdahl, 1981).

The advantages of graphic methods are offset by serious limitations. For one thing, by altering slightly the assumptions underlying a diagram, it is possible to produce an almost unlimited number of diagrams each conveying a dramatically different picture of the network. Also, as the number of members and the number of connections between members increase, interpretation of the diagram becomes increasingly difficult. For large, densely connected networks, visual displays can be so complex that they confuse understanding of the network's structure.

Related to the problem of interpretation is the difficulty of producing graphs of large networks. Traditionally, network sociograms were drawn by hand. Such approaches are more like an art form than an advanced analysis technique. There are few generally accepted procedures for developing such graphic presentations. Even with the advances in computer graphics, large complex network graphs have been slow to evolve. In some cases, plotting programs developed for other purposes have been used to create graphic depictions of networks. But since these programs were not designed to provide visual images of networks, they often have serious limitations when applied to network data (Klovdahl, 1986).[2] Graph models of organizational relations are presented and discussed in Gillespie et al. (1986).

Matrix Models

Use of the matrix has become the dominant approach to network analysis in recent years. It produces algebraic representations of network relations. While a matrix does not stimulate the kind of intuitive understanding that a simple graph model does, it has nonetheless become prominent because it expresses all the information pictured in a graph model. Moreover, it also facilitates more extensive quantitative analyses.

A matrix presents a network in the form of an array of units arranged in rows and columns. In a typical network matrix, the rows represent network members and the columns represent the same set of members in identical sequence. Each cell in the matrix contains a number which represents the relationship between two members of the network. Usually a one represents a relationship between two members and a zero represents the absence of a relationship. Matrices can represent both directional and non-directional relations among the network members. With directional relations, the members arrayed in the matrix rows are typically treated as initiators or senders of the content in a relationship, and the members arrayed across the columns are recipients of the content in a relationship (Knoke and Kuklinski, 1982). If directional relationships in a network are not completely reciprocal, the matrix is asymmetrical. That is, the number in row i and column j is not identical to the number in the row j and column i. The matrix is symmetrical when directional relationships are reciprocal, or when the data represents non-directional relationships. Then, the number for every link from i to j is also represented in the link from j to i. Table 2 shows two hypothetical matrices, one symmetrical and the other asymmetrical.

The networks represented by each matrix in Table 2 are comprised of five units, A through E. The presence of a 1 in a cell indicates that a relationship exists between the two members represented by the cell's coordinates; a zero indicates no relationship. Rows represent senders and columns represent recipients. Each matrix contains twenty-five cells (N^2), and each matrix also contains ten ones. In the symmetrical matrix, however, all relationships are reciprocal; relations between the two members go both directions. For example, A has a relationship directed at B and B in turn has a relationship directed at A. In the asymmetrical matrix, only the relationship between D and E is reciprocal. All others are non-reciprocal or directional relationships. For example, B sends something to A but A does not send anything to B.

Network Partitioning. The matrix approach is especially appropriate for analyzing structural properties in networks. As shown in Table 1, such analyses can focus on the individual member, subgroups within the total network, or the total network. While all three levels of analysis are useful, there has been growing

Table 2

Hypothetical Symmetrical and Asymmetrical Matrices
for a Network of Five Members

		Symmetrical Relations							Asymmetrical Relations				
				Receive							Receive		
		A	B	C	D	E			A	B	C	D	E
Send	A	0	1	0	0	1	Send	A	0	0	0	1	1
	B	1	0	1	0	0		B	1	0	0	0	0
	C	0	1	0	0	1		C	0	1	0	1	1
	D	0	0	0	0	1		D	0	1	0	0	1
	E	1	0	1	1	0		E	0	1	0	1	0

attention placed on partitioning total networks into subgroups. This trend has been facilitated in part by the development of computer software which makes it possible to manipulate larger matrices (Burt, 1989; MacEvoy and Freeman, 1987). Early methods of detecting subgroups focused on small groups and used overly stringent criteria (Festinger, 1949; Luce and Perry, 1949). More recently, criteria of structural equivalence have been developed which subsume the earlier clique detection methods and apply well to larger networks (Burt, 1977).

Structural equivalence takes into account the pattern of connections among all members of the total network. Unlike the early clique detection methods which were based on relations among members of the subgroup, this approach detects subgroups based on their similar patterns of relations with other members of the network. In other words, members are grouped in a structurally equivalent group when they have comparable patterns of linkages with other members of the network, even if they do not maintain relations with one another (Lorrain and White, 1971).

Central to structural equivalence analysis is the concept of distance. Using the structural equivalence criterion, distance between network members is measured by the degree of similarity in their patterns of interaction: the greater the similarity, the shorter the distance. If two members have exactly identical patterns with other members, their distance from each other is zero. The greater the differences in their patterns of interaction, the greater the distance between them. Even when members have no direct connection to one another, they may have small distance scores and be treated as structurally equivalent.

Once the distances between all members of the network have been established, the members are assigned to structurally equivalent groups using one of two methods of partitioning: agglomerative clustering or divisive partitioning. Agglomerative clustering analysis identifies homogeneous subgroups (Bailey, 1975; Burt, 1976; Romesburg, 1984). In the initial step of the analysis, each member is treated as a cluster. In successive steps, clusters are aggregated by combining members with similar patterns of interaction. After a cluster is identified, it is evaluated as a new unit and its distance from the other clusters is determined. This process can continue until the entire network is treated as a single cluster.

Most standard statistical packages have agglomerative clustering algorithms. An advantage of the agglomerative clustering over the divisive partitioning is that there are goodness-of-fit statistical tests to assess the extent to which a set of cases occupies a structural equivalent in the network (Burt, 1983:277). One criticism of this approach is that no standards have been established to determine when the clustering process should be stopped.

Divisive partitioning methods start with the entire network and successively divide it into smaller and smaller subgroups. Each successive step divides the network into two subsets that are distinctive and different. This is opposite of the agglomerative cluster methods where two members that are most similar are joined. Interestingly, although the most popular statistical packages include one or more agglomerative clustering algorithms, none of these packages have divisive partitioning algorithms.

The most widely used divisive partitioning method is blockmodeling (Breiger et al., 1975; White et al., 1976; Arabie et al., 1978), and the most widely used blockmodeling algorithm is called CONCOR (CONvergence of iterated CORrelations).[3] CONCOR is an iterative correlation program which processes the network matrix to produce a Pearson's r coefficient for each pair of members in the network. The larger the correlation, the greater the similarity between the two members. CONCOR next processes the matrix of correlation coefficients to produce a matrix of second-order correlations. Each successive matrix is submitted to the program until all correlations in the matrix are either +1 or -1. This result is the first partitioning of the network into two structurally equivalent groups. The process is repeated on each block until the desired number of subgroups is obtained.

The primary distinction between agglomerative and divisive methods is their assumption about space. Blockmodeling classifies network members into discrete, mutually exclusive and exhaustive categories. It does not produce measures of distance between the blocks or any ordering of the relationships among the blocks. Cluster analysis, on the other hand, preserves distance measures during the aggregation process. This makes it possible to apply statistical methods for testing hypotheses (Burt, 1980).

CONCOR has been criticized as lacking validation. That is, there is no proof that convergence of the correlation matrix actually represents structurally equivalent positions. This is in contrast to the goodness-of-fit tests available with the agglomerative clustering techniques. It is also unclear what objective function is minimized or maximized by the process (Schwartz, 1977). On the other hand, its proponents argue that it has been found to consistently produce interpretable blocks (Arabie and Boorman, 1982).

ANALYSIS OF AN INTERORGANIZATIONAL NETWORK

The data for this analysis originate from a population of 80 emergency service organizations (Gillespie et al., 1986). These organizations constitute a significant part of the social service delivery network that would aid the surrounding metropolitan area in the event of a natural disaster. To identify this network, contacts were made with over 900 social service organizations. Of those 900 organizations, 84 (9%) indicated that they would provide emergency services in response to an earthquake. Officials of each organization were identified as key informants for the study. Three follow-up mailings of a questionnaire to these informants were carried out at approximately three week intervals. Informants who did not respond to the mailings were telephoned again, and in a few cases visits were made to the agency to meet with them. The final set of 80 emergency service organizations represents 95% of the acknowledged emergency social service agency population during the summer of 1985.

The questionnaire was designed to illicit information about each organization and its relationships with other organizations both under normal day-to-day operations and during the first 24 to 48 hours after an earthquake. In order to obtain data on both normal operations and the postdisaster response period, an earthquake scenario was presented in the questionnaire. While it would be preferable to observe the network under actual disaster conditions, the scenario methodology provides a common referent for all informants and eliminates the need to wait until a disaster strikes before studying the network. This methodology is also consistent with a common approach used in predisaster planning activities where scenarios provide the basis for training exercises and simulations (Mileti et al., 1981; Belardo et al., 1983; Congressional Research Service, 1984; Wallace and DeBalogh, 1985). To make the scenario as realistic as possible, it was written to be consistent with the empirical damage assessment literature, as well as the opinions of local emergency management officials (Gillespie et al., 1986).

Preliminary Analysis

As a first step in the analysis, two 93 by 93 matrices were constructed representing linkages between members for both the pre and postdisaster periods. These matrices consist of the original 80 organizations in the study, plus 13 additional organizations which were cited as being important to the organizations in the original study. In order to be added to the matrix, an organization must have been listed by at least two other organizations in the original network of 80 organizations.

Preliminary analysis of this network indicated that one organization, the American Red Cross, appeared to be the most central in the network. This organization had a total of 43 direct connections to other members of the network across the pre and postdisaster networks. This compares with 26 and 25 for the Salvation Army and the County Office of Civil Preparedness respectively, the next two most central organizations in the network. For this analysis, it was decided to focus only on the organization set of the American Red Cross (ARC) which includes all the other network members with which it has direct ties (Aldrich and Whetten, 1981).

Focusing on the ARC organization set is a reasonable first step in the process of partitioning the total network into subparts. It has been noted that organization sets, or "ego-networks" represent the simplest level of network analysis (Burt, 1982). Limiting the analysis to the organization set brings into sharper focus the patterns of interaction around one of the central actors in the total network. It has also been pointed out that of all possible units of analysis within social networks, organization sets are the most likely unit of analysis to show change over time or under different conditions (Burt, 1983). In addition, the concept of organization set has important ties to the earliest interorganizational theories (Evan, 1966; Caplow, 1964).

On the practical side, the organization set is consistent with our initial perceptions about the structure of the network. The ARC is a dual purpose organization, being involved in both emergency preparedness and more traditional social services. Therefore, it might be expected to act as a linking organization for the social service units and the government emergency management units in the total network. In addition, our initial analysis indicated that the ARC's organization set contained all of the most significant organizations in the total network. Finally, the ARC organization set is a smaller subset of the total network which makes the analysis more manageable and easier to understand.

The ARC organization set is comprised of 44 organizations, the ARC and the 43 organizations with which it has direct ties across the pre and postdisaster networks. Each member of the network is identified as having primarily a social service or emergency management function. Twenty-six of the members of the ego-network were identified as social service organizations and 18 were found to be emergency management organizations.

Identifying Structurally Equivalent Positions

STRUCTURE, Version 4.1, was used to partition the ARC's organization set into structurally equivalent groups known as positions in the network. STRUCTURE uses hierarchical agglomerative cluster analysis to identify clusters of network members which have similar patterns of interaction with other members of the network. As noted earlier, these members do not necessarily have to be connected directly or indirectly to one another. Such clusters represent positions in a network which are said to be structurally equivalent. STRUCTURE evaluates each position by producing reliability scores for each member and an overall position reliability score. The member scores indicate how well each case fits with the other cases in the cluster. The position reliability score is an indicator of how well the cluster, taken as a whole, meets the criteria of structural equivalence. This reliability derives from a principal component analysis which yields the ratio of variance accounted for by the first principal component to the total variance (Burt, 1983:277-278).

The goal of structural equivalence analysis is to simplify the structure of relations in a network so that it is possible to understand the various kinds and patterns of interactions occurring in the network. Therefore, it is most useful to produce a small number of highly reliable groups. On the other hand, achieving the highest possible reliability may differentiate otherwise similar clusters, which increases the number of groups and shows a more complex structure than necessary or desirable. It is thus important to strike a balance between the criterion of high reliability and the criterion of a manageable number of clusters. Our experience indicates that somewhere between two and six clusters provide a reasonable summary of the network, and three or four is perhaps most useful. Still, it is important to keep in mind that no set prescription for analysis will fit every network. The number of groups and the level of reliability must be dictated by the unique circumstances of any analysis.

Producing structurally equivalent groups using STRUCTURE is a two step process. First, STRUCTURE performs a cluster analysis of the network matrix. Output from this analysis is then used to identify clusters and to test member and position reliability. As pointed out above, one of the criticisms of cluster analysis is that no standards have been established to determine when the clustering process should be stopped. Therefore, it is necessary for the researcher to develop a protocol for developing and testing structurally equivalent positions. See Appendix I for a description of the testing protocol used in the present example.

As shown in Table 3, applying the testing protocol to the ARC organization set produced six structurally equivalent positions in the predisaster network, with each position including between 4 and 13 organizations. In addition, the ARC represents a single, additional, unique position in the network.[4] Position 6 contains eight organizations which are not tied to any other organization in the predisaster network and this position is therefore a group of isolates in the network. Since no member of this group is tied to any other member of the network, the overall group reliability score is 1.00, even though they are not connected to the network. Reliability scores for the other five positions ranged from .76 to .94. There is no way to calculate reliability for the ARC because it holds a single unique position in the network.

In the postdisaster network, only one structurally equivalent group was produced which achieved a reliability of over .80. That group contains forty-one organizations with a position reliability of .81. As in the predisaster network, the ARC was identified as a single organization representing a unique position in the network. In addition, two other organizations also occupied unique positions, the Salvation Army and the County Office of Civil Preparedness. Like the ARC, they serve unique functions by providing multiple linkages to the one structurally equivalent group. If we look at those two organizations individually, we see that one of them, the Salvation Army, is a key actor in the social service system. The other, the County Office of Civil Preparedness, is a key actor in the emergency management system. It is likely that all three of the organizations (the ARC, Salvation Army, and the County Office of Civil Preparedness) represent central actors in the postdisaster network. One of the weaknesses of the STRUCTURE program is that it does not allow adequate analysis of such single-member positions which serve significant functions in the network.

These structural configurations show that the pre- and post-disaster networks are quite different in their patterns of interaction. An important difference relates to the role of emergency management and social service organizations. Table 3 shows the number of social service and emergency management organizations in each position for the pre and postdisaster networks.

Table 3

Number of Social Service and Emergency Management Organizations in Each Structurally Equivalent Position in the Pre and Postdisaster Networks

	Social Service	Emergency Management	Total
Predisaster Network:			
Position 1	0	7	7
Position 2	2	4	6
Position 3	13	0	13
Position 4	3	1	4
Position 5	5	0	5
Position 6	6	2	8
Red Cross	1		1
Postdisaster Network:			
Position 1	24	17	41
Red Cross	1		1
Salvation Army	1		1
Co. Civil Prep.		1	1

Table 3 shows that in the predisaster network there are six structurally equivalent positions dominated by either social service or emergency management organizations. This indicates that under normal conditions barriers exist between social service and emergency management organizations in this network. This is a strikingly different pattern from the postdisaster network where nearly all organizations fit into a single group, regardless of their organizational type. In the postdisaster condition, the normal lines of differentiation break down as all members of the network focus their interaction to facilitate a more effective response to the disaster.

Relations Between Structurally Equivalent Positions

After the network is partitioned into structurally equivalent positions, patterns of relations within and between the positions are examined using two summary matrices: a block density matrix and an image matrix (Burt, 1982; Knoke and Kuklinski, 1982). A density matrix shows the proportion of potential linkages that are actually sent from a row position to a column position. It is possible for a position to send many linkages to other positions and not receive linkages in return. Another possibility is for a position to be internally linked, with members of the block sending links to one another.

An image matrix simplifies the original matrix by replacing the density scores with either a 1 or 0 depending on the relative magnitudes of the densities (White et al., 1976). If the density exceeds a predetermined cutoff criteria, a 1 is placed in the image matrix cell, otherwise the cell is given a 0. In our analysis the overall average density scores for the complete pre and postdisaster matrices are used as a cutoff criteria for the image matrices.

Table 4 shows position density and image matrices for the pre and postdisaster networks. Each cell in the density matrix indicates the proportion of linkages which exist between members of each row structurally equivalent position and each column position. In the postdisaster density matrix, several of the scores are 1.00. This means that each of the single unique organizations in the network are connected to one another. Because they represent single organizations rather than groupings of organizations, a 1.00 appears in the matrix if the organizations are connected and a .00 appears if there is no connection between the two organizations.

In the predisaster network, scores in the density matrix range from .00 to .95. In the postdisaster network, the scores range from .00 to .94. For example, in the predisaster network, position 1 is strongly linked to itself because 68% (.68 × 100) of all the possible linkages between the organizations in position 1 are actually found to exist. In contrast, for the postdisaster network, only 8% of all possible linkages between the members of position 1 are present.

Using the predisaster network to illustrate, the overall density score of .21 is used for the cut off point. For density scores greater than the overall average density value, the corresponding cell in the image matrix is given a 1. The image matrix shows that five positions are internally linked in the predisaster condition. In addition, several of the positions send enough linkages to other positions to produce density scores greater that the overall score of .21. The image matrix for the postdisaster network was constructed in the same manner, using .12 as the cutoff criteria.

Comparing the pre and postdisaster density and image matrices illustrates why it is important to produce a relatively small number of structurally equivalent groups. As pointed out above, the larger the number of structurally equivalent groups produced using STRUCTURE, the more difficult it is to present the results graphically and interpret them. In this case, we could have simplified the matrices by eliminating the 8 organizations in position 6 from the predisaster network since they are not connected to the network under normal conditions. However, this would have created additional problems of interpretation because the pre and postdisaster networks would not have contained the same organizations.

Two additional image matrices were derived from the original matrices presented in Table 4. Table 5 shows domination and coalition matrices for the pre and postdisaster networks (Breiger, 1976; DiMaggio, 1986). In the Domination matrix, a 1 is placed in the cell if the row position receives in the original density matrix a greater proportion of its links from the column position than the proportion it sends (remember the matrix convention of rows as the sender and

Table 4

Density and Image Matrices for Structurally Equivalent Positions in the Pre and Post Disaster Networks.

Predisaster Network

Density Matrix

	1	2	3	4	5	6	ARC
1	.68	.34	.10	.39	.37	.00	.79
2	.34	.51	.11	.48	.50	.00	.95
3	.07	.09	.47	.38	.60	.00	.40
4	.19	.29	.17	.29	.38	.00	.94
5	.11	.17	.27	.22	.46	.00	.81
6	.00	.00	.00	.00	.00	.00	.00
ARC	.33	.50	.12	.50	.50	.00	.00

Image Matrix

	1	2	3	4	5	6	ARC
1	1	1	0	1	1	0	1
2	1	1	0	1	1	0	1
3	0	0	1	1	1	0	1
4	0	1	0	1	1	0	1
5	0	0	1	1	1	0	1
6	0	0	0	0	0	0	0
ARC	1	1	0	1	1	0	0

Overall Average Density: .21

Postdisaster Network

Density Matrix*

	1	ARC	SA	CODP
1	.08	.94	.54	.40
ARC	.07	.00	1.00	1.00
SA	.26	1.00	.00	1.00
COCP	.25	1.00	1.00	.00

Image Matrix

	1	ARC	SA	CODP
1	0	1	1	1
ARC	0	0	1	1
SA	1	1	0	1
COCP	1	1	1	0

Overall Average Density: .12

*The postdisaster network produced 1 large structurally equivalent position and 3 single unique organizations. Therefore, the density scores for these organizations do not represent the proportion of linkages between them but whether or not a linkage exists.

columns as recipients). In the coalition matrix, a 1 appears in the cell if the row and column positions send linkages reciprocally to one another.

Looking first at the Domination matrices, we see evidence of domination in both the pre and postdisaster network. In the predisaster network, position 4 and position 5 are dominant over position 1, position 4 and the ARC are dominant over position 3, and position 5 is dominant over position 2. This pattern of domination is diffuse, indicating no strong domination by any single actor or group in the predisaster network. In the postdisaster network, the ARC emerges as dominant over position 1 which contains 41 of the 43 other members of the network.

The Coalition matrix shows a complex pattern of coalition among the structurally equivalent groups in the predisaster condition. Five of the six positions represent individual coalitions because of the high concentration of interaction among the members of each position. In addition, two clusters of organizations form identifiable coalitions. Position 1 and position 2 appear to form one coalition and position 3, position 4 and position 5 form another. The

Table 5
Patterns of Domination and Coalition in the Pre and Postdisaster Networks

PreDisaster Network

Domination Matrix

	1	2	Positions 3	4	5	6	ARC
1	0	0	0	1	1	0	0
2	0	0	0	0	1	0	0
3	0	0	0	1	0	0	1
4	0	0	0	0	0	0	0
5	0	0	0	0	0	0	0
6	0	0	0	0	0	0	0
ARC	0	0	0	0	0	0	0

Coalition Matrix

	1	2	Positions 3	4	5	6	ARC
1	1	1	0	0	0	0	1
2	1	1	0	1	0	0	1
3	0	0	1	0	1	0	0
4	0	1	0	1	1	0	1
5	0	0	1	1	1	0	1
6	0	0	0	0	0	0	0
ARC	1	1	0	1	1	0	0

PostDisaster Network

Domination Matrix

	1	ARC	SA	COCP
1	0	1	0	0
ARC	0	0	0	0
SA	0	0	0	0
COCP	0	0	0	0

Coalition Matrix

	1	ARC	SA	COCP
1	0	0	1	1
ARC	0	0	1	1
SA	1	1	0	1
COCP	1	1	1	0

ARC, holding its unique position linking the network, has coalition relations with 4 of the 6 groups: position 1, position 2, position 4, and position 5.

In the postdisaster network, position 1 and two of the unique single organizations, Salvation Army and the County Office of Civil Preparedness, appear to comprise a coalition. The ARC does not maintain coalition relations with the one large group in the postdisaster network. Rather, as the domination matrix shows, the ARC is dominant over this group. The ARC does, however, maintain coalition relations with the Salvation Army and the County Office of Civil Preparedness.

These domination and coalition matrices indicate the importance of exploring different patterns of interaction in order to understand the structure of a network. By examining only the domination matrix, we might conclude that in the predisaster network no organization assumes a dominant position over all or most other members of the network. In the postdisaster network, we would note that the ARC is dominant over a position which contains nearly all members of the network. On the other hand, if we had only examined the coalition matrices, we might conclude that the ARC is tied to several coalitions in the predisaster network but is connected only to the Salvation Army and County Office of Civil Preparedness in the postdisaster network. By constructing both the domination and coalition matrices, we are able to gain a better understanding of the overall network and, in this case, an understanding of how it changes from pre to postdisaster conditions.

For example, it appears that the postdisaster network has a much more concentrated pattern of relations. The ARC is perhaps the most central actor in the network, yet the other two residual organizations also have important roles with patterns of interaction which are unique and unlike those of the other organizations in the network. All three residual organizations are central to the network.

Integrating Network Analysis with More Traditional Analyses

To this point, the analysis has focused on the structure of the predisaster and postdisaster networks. Network analysis can also be used in conjunction with conventional forms of analysis. For example, it is possible to develop descriptive profiles of the structurally equivalent positions by examining mean scores for key characteristics of the members of each position. When using this type of analysis, one must be cautious in comparing profiles across conditions, such as the pre and postdisaster networks used in our analysis, because the composition and size of the groups may vary greatly in the different networks. This is especially a problem for the postdisaster network because it is comprised almost entirely of one large structurally equivalent group. For this reason we will only present profiles for the predisaster network.

Table 6 presents a descriptive profile of each predisaster network position using means for selected organizational variables. Variables included in the table are: level of disaster preparedness, capacity to respond to different types of disasters, capacity to provide a variety of disaster relevant services, previous experience in disaster response, and degree of organizational formalization.

These positions in the predisaster network show considerable variation in the selected organizational characteristics. Position 1 and position 6 appear to have higher means on most variables than the other groups. They show lower mean values only on previous experience. No test was performed to determine if there is a statistically significant difference between the groups because of the large differences in group size. However, if a network analysis does produce roughly equivalent sized groups and the variables meet the assumptions for the statistics used, it would be appropriate to test for significance of the difference between the means of the various groups.

CONCLUSIONS

Relations between units are basic to all conceptualizations of social systems (Hall and Fagen, 1956). Approaches to understanding social systems, such as general systems theory, have been criticized for high levels of abstraction and operational inadequacy (Buckley, 1968). Network analysis can be used to overcome these difficulties by specifying and operationalizing basic aspects of the relations in a social system.

Table 6

Mean Values on Selected Organizational Characteristics for the Structural Equivalent Positions in the Predisaster Network

Positions	1	2	3	4	5	6
Preparedness	2.08	1.42	0.65	1.54	1.21	1.74
Disaster Capacity	6.88	5.01	3.18	5.59	5.33	5.88
Service Capacity	4.46	4.04	2.12	3.38	4.32	5.17
Experience	0.67	0.74	0.49	0.82	1.23	0.54
Formalization	3.07	2.88	2.53	2.50	2.67	3.02

Overall measures of network relations provide descriptions of both the content and form of social systems. The size of a network, its connectedness (density), centrality, formalization, and hierarchy reflect important social conditions. These measures provide information on context and thus give an important foundation upon which to study system structure and processes. In addition, partitioning network relations into systems can reveal modes of operation and establish patterns of interdependency. Descriptions of subgroups and the relations between subgroups offer great potential for documenting situational determinants and contingencies in theory. The opportunity to examine system-subsystem relations is of particular importance because theorists claim that most of the variance at one level is accounted for by variance at the next higher level of analysis (Hage, 1980).

Each of the different techniques used in network analysis have advantages and disadvantages. Graphic depictions of unit-specific relations provide useful overall impressions (Gillespie et al., 1986). Such impressions facilitate an intuitive understanding of networks. The disadvantage is that these descriptions are static and limited to single variable accounts. More abstract graphic depictions based on types of units or social roles provide greater generalizability and also allow the researcher greater control in illustrating aspects of the network. The disadvantage here is that graphs are complicated to interpret and the aggregation process requires a great deal of time and effort to develop and implement.

Blockmodel and cluster analysis offer alternative methods for discovering homogeneous subgroups within networks. Both are complicated and difficult to interpret. Nevertheless both are valuable because they offer a window into the data which can help advance causal models of complex social systems. Subgroups within networks represent one of the primary building blocks in social theory. The measures of network relations which are produced with various cluster analyses represent basic features of social systems. Partitioning of overall density relations into the specific density relations among structurally equivalent positions can reveal the most dramatic changes in these relationships.

Network analysis is most effective when combined with other methods in developing theory. Identifying clusters and blocks, or observing patterns in graphic models are techniques which enhance descriptions of members' behavior and the systems within which the behavior takes place. Finally, testing hypotheses about networks requires comparable data from many networks, or large networks with many subgroups so that the output from network analysis may be imported into standard data files for conventional quantitative analyses.

REFERENCE NOTES

1. For example, Burt (1982) develops a sixfold typology of network analysis by cross-classifying two analytic approaches with three levels of analysis. Burt's typology provides useful guidelines to the range of procedures subsumed in network analysis.

2. An interactive graphics program called VIEW_NET is now available which is designed especially for network analyses. VIEW_NET is a menu-drive program which can handle networks up to 2000 members. For an introduction to VIEW_NET, see Klovdahl (1986).

3. Other discrete distance methods and computer algorithms may be found in Edwards and Cavalli-Sforza (1965), Friedman and Rubin (1967), and Hartigan (1975).

4. STRUCTURE produces structurally equivalent groups and a residual category of units which do not fit in any group. In this analysis, the ARC remained in the residual category because its patterns of interaction were different from any other organization in the network. However, it should be noted that some residual units carry out unique roles in the network, as the case here where the ARC is the central organization in the network.

REFERENCES

Aldenderfer, M.S. and R.K. Blashfield. 1984. *Cluster Analysis.* Beverly Hills, California: Sage Publications Inc.

Aldrich, H. and D.A. Whetten. 1981. "Organization-sets, action-sets, and networks: making the most of simplicity." In P. Nystrom and W. Starbuck (Editors), *Handbook of Organization Design*, Volume 1. London: Oxford University Press.

Arabie, P., Boorman, S. A., & Levitt, P. R. (1978). "Constructing blockmodels: How and why." *Journal of Mathematical Psychology*, 17, 21-63.

Arabie, P. & Boorman, S. A. (1982). "Blockmodel: developments and perspectives." In H. Hudson (Ed.), *Classifying Social Data: New Applications of Analytic Methods for Social Science Research*. San Francisco: Jossey-Bass.

Bailey, K. (1975). "Cluster Analysis." In D. R. Heise (Ed.), *Sociological Methodology* (pp. 59-128). San Francisco: Jossey-Bass.

Belardo, S., Pazer, H. L., Wallace, W. A. & Danko, W. D. (1983). "Simulation of a crisis management information network: A serendipitous evaluation." *Decision Science*, 14, 588-606.

Bott, E. (1955) "Urban Families: Conjugal Roles and Social Networks." *Human Relations*, 8, 345-383.

Breiger, R. L. (1976). "Career attributes and network structure: A blockmodel of a biomedical research specialty." *American Sociological Review*, 41, 117-135.

Breiger, R. L., Boorman, S. A., & P. Arabie. (1975). "An algorithm for clustering relational data, with application to social network analysis and comparison to multi-dimensional scaling." *Journal of Mathematical Psychology*, 12, 328-383.

Buckley, W. (1968). *Modern Systems Research for the Behavioral Scientist*. Chicago: Aldine.

Burt, R. S. (1989). *STRUCTURE, Version 4.1*. New York: Research Center in Structural Analysis, Columbia University.

Burt, R. S. (1983). "Cohesion Versus Structural Equivalence as a Basis for Network Subgroups." In R. S. Burt and M. K. Minor (Eds.). *Applied Network Analysis: A Methodological Introduction*. Beverly Hills: Sage Publications, Inc.

Burt, R. S. (1982). *Toward a Structural Theory of Action*. New York: Academic Press.

Burt, R. S. (1980). "Models of network structure." In A. Inkeles, J. Coleman and N. Smelser (Eds.), *Annual Review of Sociology*, 6, 79-101.

Burt, R.S. (1977). "Positions in Multiple Network Systems. Part One: A General Conception of Stratification and Prestige in a System of Actors Cast as a Social Typology." *Social Forces*, 57, 106-131.

Burt, R. S. (1976). "Positions in social networks." *Social Forces*, 55, 93-122.

Caplow, T. (1964). *Principles of Organization*. Cambridge, Massachusetts: Harcourt, Brace and World.

Congressional Research Service. (1984). *Information Technology and Emergency Management*. Washington, D.C.: U.S. Government Printing Office.

DiMaggio, P. (1986) "Structural analysis of organizational fields: A blockmodel approach." *Research in Organizational Behavior*, 8, 335-370.

Edwards, A.W.F., & Cavalli-Sforza, L. (1965). "A method for cluster analysis." *Biometrics*, 21, 362-375.

Evan, W.M. (1966). "The organization-set: toward a theory of interorganizational relations." In J.D. Thompson (Editor), *Approaches to Organizational Design*. Pittsburgh: University of Pittsburgh Press.

Festinger, L. (1949). "The analysis of sociogram using matrix algebra." *Human Relations*, 2, 153-158.

Friedman, H. P. and J. Rubin. (1967). "On Some Invariant Criteria for Grouping Data." *Journal of the American Statistical Association*, 62, 1159-1178.

Gillespie, D. F., Sherraden, M. W., Streeter, C. L. and Zakour, M. J. (1986). *Mapping Networks of Organized Volunteers for Natural Hazard Preparedness*, #PB87-182051/A09. Springfield, Virginia: National Technical Information Service.

Hage, G. (1980). *Theories of Organizations: Form, Process and Transformation*. New York: John Wiley & Sons.

Hall, A. & Fagen, R. (1956). "Definition of System." *General Systems* 1, 18-28. Also appears in Buckley (Ed.), *Modern Systems Research for the Behavioral Scientist*. Chicago: Aldine Publishing Company, 1968:81-92.

Hartigan, J. A. (1975). *Clustering Algorithms*. New York: Wiley.

Klovdahl, A. S. (1986). "VIEW_NET: A new tool for network analysis." *Social Networks*, 8, 313-342.

Klovdahl, A. S. (1981). "A note on images of networks." *Social Networks*, 3, 197-214.

Knoke, D. & Kuklinski, J. H. (1982). *Network Analysis*. Beverly Hills, CA: Sage Publications.

Lorr, M. (1983). *Cluster Analysis for Social Scientists*. San Francisco: Jossey-Bass.

Lorrain, F. & White, H.C. (1971). "Structure of Individuals in Social Networks." *Journal of Mathematical Sociology*, 1, 49-80.

Luce, R. D. & Perry, A. D. (1949). "A method of matrix analysis of group structure." *Psychometrika*, 14, 95-116.

MacEvoy, B. & Freeman, L. (1987). *UCINET: A Microcomputer Package for Network Analysis*. Irvine, CA: Mathematical Social Science Group, School of Social Science, University of California at Irvine.

Mileti, D. S., Hutton, J. R. & Sorenson J. H. (1981). *Earthquake Prediction Response and Options for Public Policy*. Boulder, CO: Institute of Behavioral Science, The University of Colorado.

Moreno, J. L. (1934). *Who Shall Survive? Foundations of Sociometry, Group Psychology, and Sociodrama*. Washington D.C.: Nervous and Mental Disease Monograph, No. 58.

Paulson, S. K. (1985). "A paradigm for the analysis of interorganizational networks." *Social Networks*, 7, 105-12.

Romesburg, H.C. 1984. *Cluster Analysis for Researchers*. Belmont, California: Lifetime Learning Publications.

Schwartz, J. E. (1977). "An examination of CONCOR and related methods for blocking sociometric data." In D. R. Heise (Ed.), *Sociological Methodology* (pp. 255-282). San Francisco: Jossey-Bass.

Tichy, N. M. & Fombrun, C. (1979). "Network analysis in organizational settings." *Human Relations*, 32, 923-965.

Wallace, W. A. & DeBalogh, F. (1985). "Decision support for disaster management." *Public Administration Review*, 45, 134-146.

White, H. C., Boorman, A. & Breiger R. L. (1976). "Social structure from multiple networks: Blockmodels of roles and positions." *American Journal of Sociology*, 81, 730-780.

APPENDIX I

PROTOCOL FOR DEVELOPING AND TESTING STRUCTURALLY EQUIVALENT POSITIONS

Our protocol for testing the structurally equivalent positions begins with the dendrogram (or icicle plot) produced from the cluster analysis. STRUCTURE produces two graphs, one using distance scores based on the single-linkage method (also known as minimum method or nearest neighbor method) and the other using Ward's method (also known as minimum variance method). In this case we report on Ward's method because the single-linkage method typically resulted in chaining (Aldenderfer and Blashfield, 1984). Ward's method, however, produced distinct clusters (Romesburg, 1984). Also, Ward's method has been found to outperform other methods when clusters are well separated (Lorr, 1983). Ward's method joins cases or clusters such that there is a minimum increase in the error sums of squares for within-cluster deviations about the cluster mean. The distance between two clusters is the ANOVA sums of squares between the clusters. At each iteration stage, the within-cluster sums of squares is minimized over all partitions obtainable by merging two clusters from the previous stage. Iterations continue until all cases are merged into one cluster.

Taking the graph produced by STRUCTURE as the point of departure, lines are drawn on the output to indicate approximately the number of positions sought or reflected in the graph. If all cases are to be included, draw the line at the smallest maximum distance scores which include all cases. If it is not desirable to include all cases, make sure that "residual" cases are not central or in some other way important to the structure of the network. The lines drawn through the graph make it possible to identify clusters of members which have small distance scores.

STRUCTURE requires that three cases be selected from the network to initiate the first structurally equivalent group. Cases clustered together because of their high similarity have the likelihood of strong structural equivalence. The three middle cases in the strongest cluster are assigned to the first group or position. Individual reliabilities are tested, and if all cases have reliability scores of .80 or greater, the position reliability is tested. If the position has a reliability of .80 or higher, the next closest case is added and again the member and position reliabilities are tested. This process is continued until the reliability for one of the added cases falls below .80. When a case reliability falls below .80, remove the case and save the cluster. A cutoff of .80 was selected because it balances the reliabilities and number of positions identified, as discussed above.

This procedure is repeated until all members are included in a structurally equivalent position or no more positions can be produced which meet the minimum reliability criteria of .80. All members not included in a position should be examined individually to determine if they are strategic or unique actors in the network. If not, these members can either be dropped from the analysis or pooled together into a residual category.

Index

NOTES: *fn*–footnote; *n*–reference note; *illus.*–table or figure

Alcoholics, labeling effects on behavior of, study example 105*fn*,106-107,108,113,114, 115,117,118
Analysis of variance (ANOVA)
factorial, moderated/interaction effects testing by 170-173
interaction effects model 183-184
moderated multiple regression analysis using 173-176
multiple regression analysis models of 173

Bivariate tests, inadequacies of for categorical data analysis 106-107
BMDP software, loglinear analysis procedures 120
Burnout, worker/job, variables related to and assessment of 165-167

Canada Health Act (1984), and policy process study of 48-53
Causal inference, moderator variables' facilitation of 164,165
Child abuse/neglect
implicating factor of 60-61
parental evaluation regarding 62, 63-64. *See also* Knowledge of Normative Infant Development inventory

Child/infant development
family relations effect on 60,71, 81,82
parental knowledge of, role in 60-61
measurement of 62-64
study example of 61-62,65-83
Child welfare, and family services treatment. *See* Intensive Family Preservation Services
Classical Theory of measurement
application of, compared with alternate theories 12
applied analysis using 24,26-29
and results of, compared with alternate theories *illus.* 34; 35-36,37-38
limitations in 29
related reading 12
reliability in 17-19,37
score breakdown in 12-13
validity in 36
CONCOR software program 208, 218*n*.3
Concordance, use of in content analysis 45
Content analysis, process of 42-44, 53,56-57
computer applications toward 44-53
Contingency tests, inadequacies of for categorical data analysis 106-107

© 1992 by The Haworth Press, Inc. All rights reserved. 223

Coping, social support impact on stress and, theory regarding 180
and interaction effects of 181,182
Cox regression 132-133. *See also* Event history analysis

Data base management systems (DBMS), use in content analysis 47-53
DataEase software program, use in content analysis 48-53
Decision making, relation of to depression, theory regarding 181
and interaction effects in 181,182
and modeling of interaction effects in, example study 185-197
Depression
relation of decision making and locus of control to, theory regarding 181
and interaction effects in 181,182
and modeling of interaction effects in, example study 185-197
scale for measurement of 12
and applied comparative analysis of 24-38
Discriminant analysis
basic strategy of 97
logistic regression analysis compared to 97
time-related information in, compared with event history analysis 144, 151-152
Document analysis strategies 42-57

Environmental autonomy, relation of to personal functioning, theory regarding 181
and interaction effects of 181,183

Ethnograph software program, use in content analysis 46-47
Event history analysis
data collection implications in 154-155
and advantages of 143
and logistic regression, compared 144,151-152
method for, example study using 135-145,148-154
model and evaluator choices for 125-126,129-131,132-133, 144-145
outcome measures in, compared to logistic regression and discriminant analysis 151-154
survival function transformed to hazard rate in 126,129-133
uses for 124-125
External validity. *See* Validity

Factor analysis
confirmatory, defined 70
example study 70-81
exploratory, distinguished from confirmatory 70
example study 66-70
Failure-time analysis. *See* Event history analysis
Family relations
and child development, effect on 60,71,81,82
measurements to assess 62,64
Family services. *See* Intensive Family Preservation Services

Gender, as moderator variable, examples 165,167-168, 169,170
General Inquirer software program, use in content analysis 44-45
Generalizability Theory (G-theory) of measurement
application of 12

applied analysis using 29,31-33
comparison to Classical
Theory 33-35
results of analysis, compared
with alternate theories *illus.*
34; 35-36,37-38
related reading 12
reliability in 21-24, *illus.* 25
score breakdown in 14-17, *illus.*
18
validity in 36
Generalized Contentment Scale 12
and measurement theories'
analyses using 24-38

HOMEBUILDERS program,
services of 134-135,154.
See also Intensive Family
Preservation Services
Hospital discharge planning,
Medicare patients study
example 88-102

Index of Family Relations scale 62, 64
Index of Parental Attitudes scale
62,64
Infant development. *See* Child
development
Intensive Family Preservation
Services (IFPS)
HOMEBUILDERS program
134-135,154
analysis study of 135-145,
154. *See also* Event history
analysis
related reading 123*fn*, 124*fn*
Interaction effects, defined 160. *See also* Moderator variables
modeling of 183-185
example study 185-197
theoretical forms of 180-183
Item Response Theory of
measurement
application of 12

applied analysis using 24,
26-29
results of, compared with
alternate theories *illus.* 34;
35-36,37-38
related reading 11*fn,* 12
reliability in 19-21
score breakdown in 13-14
validity in 36

Job burnout, variables related to and
assessment of 165-167
Joint effect 160. *See also* Interaction
effects

Key word in context concordance,
use in content analysis 45
Knowledge of Normative Infant
Development (KNID)
inventory
construct validity examination
scales in 62,63-64
development of 60-61,62-63
questionnaire and study support
material, source for 59*fn*
related reading 59*fn*
study methods in 61-64
and study results 65-83

Labeling theory, study example of,
with loglinear analysis
applied to 106-107,108,
113,114,115,117,118
publication source for study
example 105*fn*
Likelihood. *See* Maximum
Likelihood Estimation
LISCOMP software program, use in
exploratory factor analysis 66
LISREL (Linear Structural
Relations)
for estimation of model
parameters 74
in interaction model tests 175

PRELIS output reading by 73
in structural equation modeling 71
uses for, additional 9
Locus of control, relation of to
depression, theory
regarding 181
and interaction effects in 181,182
and modeling of interaction effects
in, example study 185-197
LOGIST IV software program 24
source for 38*n*.5
Logistic regression
assumptions of 89-90
dependent variable to be
estimated 90-91
estimating model to fit dependent
variable 92
interpreting estimated parameters
93-95
literature review of use of 97-101
testing of model 95-96
time-related information in,
compared with event history
analysis 144, 151-152
when to use 88, 96-97
Logit analysis, loglinear model of
107-108. *See also* Loglinear
analysis
Loglinear analysis
advantages of 110-111
compared to
contingency/bivariate
testing 106-107
compared to multiple regression
107
computation of model 108-112
computational methods, reference
texts for 120-121
computer packages for 120
related reading 105*fn*
testing of models 113-118
uses for 106-108,118-120

Maximum Likelihood Estimation,
principle of 92

use of in logistic regression
92-93,95-96
Measurement issues 7
content analysis 41-57
latent variable structural equation
modeling 59-83
theories of, with comparisons
among 11-38
Moderator variables
analysis schemes for detecting
and evaluating 167-176
causal inference facilitation by
164,165
defined 160
entry of into investigative process
161-162
in interactions 162-164,180-181
and intervening variables 165-167
vs. mediated relationship, and
case example of 165-167
related reading 159*fn*,165-167
and validity threats, relation to
160-161
Multiplicative effect 160. *See also*
Interaction effects
Multivariate analytic techniques
related to quantitative
methods in social work
research 9

National Institute of Mental Health
(NIMH) Task Force on
Social Work Research, and
findings of 3-5
Networks. *See* Social networks

Parenting
effectiveness of, determinant for
60-61
effectiveness of, measures for
assessment of 61,62-64
influences on by extended family
members 151
Parent Opinion Questionnaire 62,
63-64

Index

PRELIS software program, covariance/correlation computations 73-74
Psychology, influence of on social work, and client competition 4

Qualitative variables, incorporating into quantitative analyses 7-8. *See also* specific analyses
Quantitative Methods Interest Group (QMIG) 6

Reliability, testing of model for. *See* Structural equation modeling
Regression analysis
   Cox 132-133. *See also* Event history analysis
   linear, compared to loglinear analysis 117
   logistic
     assumptions of 89-90
     dependent variable to be estimated 90-91
     estimating model to fit dependent variable 92
     interpreting estimated parameters 93-95
     literature review of use of 97-101
     testing of model 95-96
     time-related information in, compared with event history analysis 144, 151-152
     when to use 88, 96-97
   moderated multiple (MMR), interaction effects testing by 173-176
   multiple (MRA)
     ANOVA models of 173
     compared to loglinear analysis 107
     interaction effects in 184-185
     interaction effects, example study 185-197
   ordinary least squares (OLS), defined 92
     compared to logistic regression 88,92,93
     shared variance adjustment based on 168-170

SAS software program
   content analysis use of 52
   covariance/correlation computations 73-74
   logistic regression procedure, output example *illus.* 89; 92,94,95-96
   loglinear analysis procedures 120
Social networks
   analysis of
     interorganizational study 208-218
     models for 204-208
     software programs for 202,205,207,218*n*.2,218*n*.4
   properties of 202-204
Social phenomena, complex, modeling of in social work research
   event history analysis 123-155
   moderator variables in 159-176
   and interaction effects of multiple regression 179-198
   network analysis toward 213-218, 221-222
Social support, relation of to stress impact, theory regarding 180
   and interaction effects of 181,182
Social work research, criticisms of methodologies in 2-3,4-6
SPSS software program
   content analysis use of 46, 52
   covariance/correlation computations 73-74
   loglinear analysis procedures 120

Reliability subprogram, use in
    Classical Theory analysis 24
Stress, impact of, and social support
    effect on, theory regarding
    180
  and interaction effects of 181,182
Structural equation modeling/
    analysis, defined 60
  applications for 60,82-83,167-176
  confirmatory analysis type of,
    study example 70-81
  exploratory factor analysis type of
    distinguished from
    confirmatory 70
  study example 66-70
  testing of reliability and validity
    of a measure by, example
    study 60-83
STRUCTURE software program 202
  network analysis study using
    208-218,221-222
Survival analysis. *See* Event history
    analysis

Time factor in event data analysis
    125-133

Validity
  testing of a measure for. *See*
    Structural equation
    modeling
  threats to 160
  and moderator variables
    relation to 160-161
Variables
  categorical, and analysis method
    for 105-106. *See also*
    Loglinear analysis
  conditional, defined 160
  contingent, defined 160
  dependent, grouping of, strategies
    for 167-176
  dichotomous dependent, and
    statistical procedure for

    modeling 88. *See also*
      Logistic regression
  latent
    analysis strategies for 167-176
    measurement of 70,71,73
    structural equation modeling
      of 59-83
  mediating, defined 180
  moderator
    analysis schemes for detecting
      and evaluating 167-176
    causal inference facilitation by
      164,165
    defined 160
    entry of into investigative
      process 161-162
    in interactions 162-164,
      180-181
    and intervening variables
      165-167
    vs. mediated relationship, and
      case example of 165-167
    related reading 159*fn*, 165-167
    and validity threats, relation to
      160-161
  observed, measurement of latent
    variables by 70,71,73
  qualifier, defined 160
  qualitative, incorporating into
    quantitative analyses 7-8.
    See also specific analyses
  specifier, defined 160
  "third." *See* Variables, moderator
  time-varying, analysis of. *See*
    Event history analysis

Word processing programs, use in
    content analysis 45-46
Worker burnout, variables related to
    and assessment of 165-167